REDUCING BIRTH DEFECTS

MEETING THE CHALLENGE IN THE DEVELOPING WORLD

Committee on Improving Birth Outcomes
Board on Global Health

Judith R. Bale, Barbara J. Stoll, and
Adetokunbo O. Lucas, Editors

INSTITUTE OF MEDICINE
OF THE NATIONAL ACADEMIES

THE NATIONAL ACADEMIES PRESS
Washington, D.C.
www.nap.edu

THE NATIONAL ACADEMIES PRESS • 500 Fifth Street, N.W. • Washington, DC 20001

NOTICE: The project that is the subject of this report was approved by the Governing Board of the National Research Council, whose members are drawn from the councils of the National Academy of Sciences, the National Academy of Engineering, and the Institute of Medicine. The members of the committee responsible for the report were chosen for their special competences and with regard for appropriate balance.

Support for this project was provided by the Institute of Medicine. The views presented in this report are those of the Institute of Medicine Committee on Improving Birth Outcomes.

Library of Congress Cataloging-in-Publication Data

Reducing birth defects : meeting the challenge in the developing world / Committee on Improving Birth Outcomes, Board on Global Health ; Judith R. Bale, Barbara J. Stoll, and Adetokunbo O. Lucas, editors.
    p. ; cm.
Includes bibliographical references.
  ISBN 0-309-08608-6 (pbk.), 0-309-52793-7 (PDF)
  1. Abnormalities, Human—Developing countries—Prevention. 2. Maternal health services—Developing countries. 3. Pregnancy—Complications—Developing countries—Prevention. 4. Infants (Newborn)—Diseases—Developing countries—Prevention. 5. Infants (Newborn)—Developing countries—Mortality—Prevention.
  [DNLM: 1. Abnormalities—etiology. 2. Abnormalities—prevention & control. 3. Developing Countries. 4. Prenatal Care. 5. Prenatal Diagnosis. QS 675 R321 2003] I. Bale, Judith R. II. Stoll, Barbara J. III. Lucas, Adetokunbo O. IV. Institute of Medicine (U.S.). Committee on Improving Birth Outcomes.
  RG627.2.D44R438 2003
  362.19'832'091724—dc22
                         2003015499

Additional copies of this report are available from the National Academies Press, 500 Fifth Street, N.W., Lockbox 285, Washington, DC 20055; (800) 624-6242 or (202) 334-3313 (in the Washington metropolitan area); Internet, http://www.nap.edu.

For more information about the Institute of Medicine, visit the IOM home page at: www.iom.edu.

The serpent has been a symbol of long life, healing, and knowledge among almost all cultures and religions since the beginning of recorded history. The serpent adopted as a logotype by the Institute of Medicine is a relief carving from ancient Greece, now held by the Staatliche Museen in Berlin.

"Knowing is not enough; we must apply.
Willing is not enough; we must do."
—Goethe

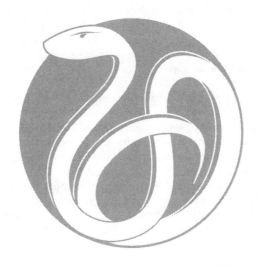

INSTITUTE OF MEDICINE
OF THE NATIONAL ACADEMIES

Shaping the Future for Health

THE NATIONAL ACADEMIES
Advisers to the Nation on Science, Engineering, and Medicine

The **National Academy of Sciences** is a private, nonprofit, self-perpetuating society of distinguished scholars engaged in scientific and engineering research, dedicated to the furtherance of science and technology and to their use for the general welfare. Upon the authority of the charter granted to it by the Congress in 1863, the Academy has a mandate that requires it to advise the federal government on scientific and technical matters. Dr. Bruce M. Alberts is president of the National Academy of Sciences.

The **National Academy of Engineering** was established in 1964, under the charter of the National Academy of Sciences, as a parallel organization of outstanding engineers. It is autonomous in its administration and in the selection of its members, sharing with the National Academy of Sciences the responsibility for advising the federal government. The National Academy of Engineering also sponsors engineering programs aimed at meeting national needs, encourages education and research, and recognizes the superior achievements of engineers. Dr. Wm. A. Wulf is president of the National Academy of Engineering.

The **Institute of Medicine** was established in 1970 by the National Academy of Sciences to secure the services of eminent members of appropriate professions in the examination of policy matters pertaining to the health of the public. The Institute acts under the responsibility given to the National Academy of Sciences by its congressional charter to be an adviser to the federal government and, upon its own initiative, to identify issues of medical care, research, and education. Dr. Harvey V. Fineberg is president of the Institute of Medicine.

The **National Research Council** was organized by the National Academy of Sciences in 1916 to associate the broad community of science and technology with the Academy's purposes of furthering knowledge and advising the federal government. Functioning in accordance with general policies determined by the Academy, the Council has become the principal operating agency of both the National Academy of Sciences and the National Academy of Engineering in providing services to the government, the public, and the scientific and engineering communities. The Council is administered jointly by both Academies and the Institute of Medicine. Dr. Bruce M. Alberts and Dr. Wm. A. Wulf are chair and vice chair, respectively, of the National Research Council.

www.national-academies.org

REVIEWERS

This report has been reviewed in draft form by individuals chosen for their diverse perspectives and technical expertise, in accordance with procedures approved by the NRC's Report Review Committee. The purpose of this independent review is to provide candid and critical comments that will assist the institution in making its published report as sound as possible and to ensure that the report meets institutional standards for objectivity, evidence, and responsiveness to the study charge. The review comments and draft manuscript remain confidential to protect the integrity of the deliberative process. We wish to thank the following individuals for their review of this report:

O.O. AKINYANJU, University of Lagos, Lagos, Nigeria
ROBERT L. BRENT, Thomas Jefferson University Medical College, Alfred duPont Hospital for Children, Wilmington, DE
MAUREEN DURKIN, Joseph L. Mailman School of Public Health, Columbia University, New York, NY
HATEM EL-SHANTI, Jordan University of Science and Technology, Irbid, Jordan
JAIME L. FRIAS, University of Southern Florida, Tampa, FL
LUIS HEREDERO, Centro Nacional de Genetica Medica, Havana, Cuba
ZHU LI, Beijing Medical University, Beijing, People's Republic of China
VICTOR B. PENCHASZADEH, Beth Israel Medical Center, New York, NY
DENIS VILJOEN, South African Institute of Medical Research, Johannesburg, South Africa
P. WASANT, Mahidol University, Bangkok, Thailand
PAUL WISE, Boston Medical Center, Boston University, Boston, MA

Although the reviewers listed above have provided many constructive comments and suggestions, they were not asked to endorse the conclusions or recommendations nor did they see the final draft of the report before its release. The review of this report was overseen by **ELAINE L. LARSON,** Columbia University, New York, New York, and by **MARY ELLEN AVERY,** Children's Hospital, Boston, Massachusetts. Appointed by the National Research Council and Institute of Medicine, they were responsible for making certain that an independent examination of this report was carried out in accordance with institutional procedures and that all review comments were carefully considered. Responsibility for the final content of this report rests entirely with the authoring committee and the institution.

Acknowledgments

The Institute of Medicine acknowledges the committee for undertaking this report and guiding it to completion while also developing the more comprehensive report, *Improving Birth Outcomes: Meeting the Challenge in the Developing World.*

The successful completion of this report has required the input of many experts. The committee thanks the researchers and public health professionals who presented papers and provided insights at the workshop held in conjunction with the first committee meeting. The committee is grateful to Joe Leigh Simpson, committee member; Eduardo Castilla, Brazil; and Arnold Christianson, South Africa, for drafting background papers that provided the starting point for this report. The committee also thanks Nicholas Wald and Bernadette Modell, United Kingdom; Enrique Gadow, Brazil; Judith Hall, Canada; and Godfrey Oakley, Noreen Goldman, and Maureen Durkin, United States, for their technical reviews and suggestions for the report. Material on rehabilitation drafted by Maureen Durkin, Nalia Khan, Molly Thorburn, and Gregory Powell for an earlier National Academies report was invaluable for this study as well.

The committee would like to thank staff and consultants in the Institute of Medicine whose contributions were instrumental to developing and producing this report: Judith Bale, who coordinated committee and other expert input, Pamela Mangu, who organized the first committee meeting, Alison Mack, who transformed report text, Mamata Kamat for dedicated research on the prevalence of specific birth defects, and Laurie Spinelli, Jason Pellmar, and Shira Fischer for their superb support, each at a different stage of the report. Also valuable in the early development of the report was research provided by Stacey Knobler, Rose Martinez, and Marjan Najafi, and the assembling of references by summer interns Kevin Crosby and Maria Vassileva. Appreciation is extended to Rona Briere for her expert editing of the report. Other staff who were instrumental in the final stages of this report include Bronwyn Schrecker, Janice Mehler (National Academies), Jennifer Otten, Jennifer Bitticks, and the NAP production staff. Andrea Cohen is acknowledged for her careful monitoring of study finances.

Contents

PREFACE   xiii

EXECUTIVE SUMMARY   1

1 INTRODUCTION   11
   Magnitude of the Problem, 12
   Increase in the Importance of Birth Defects with Decreasing
      Infant Mortality, 14
   Reducing Birth Defects in Countries with Low Infant Mortality, 15
   Social, Economic, and Health Context, 17
   Study Purpose, 18
   Study Approach, 19
   Organization of the Report, 20
   References, 20

2 IMPACT AND PATTERNS OF OCCURRENCE   22
   Genetic Birth Defects, 23
   Birth Defects of Environmental Origin, 35
   Birth Defects of Complex and Unknown Origin, 51
   Conclusion, 54
   References, 55

3 INTERVENTIONS TO REDUCE THE IMPACT OF BIRTH
   DEFECTS   68
   Basic Reproductive Care, 69
   Low-Cost Preventive Strategies, 71

Provision of Improved Care, 80
Screening for Genetic Disorders, 92
National Coordination, Surveillance, and Monitoring, 110
Conclusion, 112
References, 113

4   INCORPORATING CARE FOR BIRTH DEFECTS INTO
    HEALTH CARE SYSTEMS   122
    Strategies for Addressing Birth Defects, 122
    National Policy and Leadership, 129
    Conclusion, 133
    References, 134

APPENDIXES

A   PREVALENCE OF BIRTH DEFECTS   135
    Birth Defects, 136
    Down Syndrome, 144
    Thalassemia, 150
    Sickle Cell Disease, 154
    Glucose-6-Phosphate Dehydrogenase Deficiency, 158
    Oculocutaneous Albinism, 164
    Cystic Fibrosis, 168
    Phenylketonuria, 170
    Neural Tube Defects and Hydrocephalus, 174
    Congenital Heart Disease, 184
    Cleft Lip and/or Cleft Palate, 192
    Talipes, 202
    Developmental Dysplasia of the Hip, 206
    References, 212

B   COMMITTEE BIOGRAPHIES   220

GLOSSARY   227

ACRONYMS   239

INDEX   241

Preface

We have no trust more sacred than our children and no duty more important than providing for their health. The twentieth century saw tremendous improvements in overall child survival and well-being, yet this transformation has not been shared by all. The suffering of millions of infants who endure poverty and conflict is compounded by illness and debilitating birth defects. Even in low-resource settings, effective and affordable interventions can reduce the incidence and consequences of several major birth defects. The focus of this report is on identifying how and where such successes can be achieved in developing countries.

It is estimated that each year, more than 4 million children are born with serious birth defects that cause death or lifelong disability for the patient and hardship for entire families. Stigma, discrimination, social isolation, lost hopes and opportunities, and the daily stresses associated with lifelong impairment add to the physical and economic burdens.

To reduce the impact of birth defects, national health officials and policy makers may need first to recognize the enormous personal and societal consequences imposed by these conditions, much as they have recognized the burden of infectious diseases and acted to control them. Information on the prevalence and burden of disease caused by birth defects is scant or totally lacking in most developing countries. Such knowledge can lead to better diagnosis and treatment of birth defects, as well as to systems of care that are tailored to meet priority needs. The committee's findings and recommendations target birth defects in developing countries, where resources are limited and the needs are great. This report is intended to help focus attention on providing pregnant women the care they need and children the best possible start in life.

REDUCING BIRTH DEFECTS

MEETING THE CHALLENGE
IN THE DEVELOPING WORLD

Executive Summary

More than 4 million children are born with birth defects each year. There is little doubt that birth defects cause enormous harm in settings where risk factors for many conditions are elevated and resources for health care are limited. Yet today there is an unprecedented opportunity to prevent many birth defects and reduce the consequences of those that occur, and to do so at reasonable cost. For example, the incidence of neural tube defects can be dramatically reduced if women have an adequate intake of folic acid before and during pregnancy. This can be accomplished at low cost by fortifying a widely consumed food staple, such as wheat or corn flour. Impaired mental development due to iodine deficiency can also be prevented at relatively low cost through the iodization of salt. Congenital rubella syndrome can be prevented through the immunization of children and women. And public health education and preventive health care services can reduce the incidence of Down syndrome by discouraging childbearing in women over 35 years of age and can address the *in utero* effects of alcohol by discouraging its use during pregnancy.

Improvements in the care of children with birth defects can also be made even with limited resources. Affordable medications, surgical treatments, and community-based rehabilitation can help these children lead more normal lives. This care can be made accessible through existing primary health services, which can make referrals to, and receive support from, secondary and tertiary care facilities.

Once countries have successfully implemented basic prevention and care, screening programs for common genetic birth defects become an important mechanism for further lowering infant mortality. Genetic screening can detect risk factors associated with birth defects before conception as well as prenatally. For confirmed severe birth defects, where legal, termination of pregnancy can be offered after nondirective counseling to support each woman in the decision that is appropriate for her. Screening of newborns has the potential to improve the care of children born with treatable genetic or metabolic diseases. For neonates with phenylketonuria, early appropriate treatment has been shown effective in preventing mental retardation and other adverse health outcomes. Although such programs are significantly more expensive than the first set of interventions cited, their implementation is warranted in countries that have already reduced infant mortality from more common causes, because birth defects then become a major cause of infant mortality.

Several developing countries are making progress toward reducing infant mortality. A smaller number of developing countries with more comprehensive health care systems are also making significant progress in the prevention and care of birth defects. This report describes a variety of such programs, several in low-income settings. In many developing countries, policy makers have limited knowledge of the negative impact of birth defects and are largely unaware of the affordable and effective interventions to prevent these conditions. This report presents a plan of action to address critical gaps in the understanding, prevention, and treatment of birth defects in developing countries.

BACKGROUND AND SCOPE OF THE STUDY

Despite important advances in the prevention and treatment of several birth defects, their incidence and impact remain high in most developing countries. As neonatal mortality falls, birth defects account for an increasing proportion of infant deaths. This study addresses the prevention of birth defects and the care provided to children with birth defects by:

- Reviewing current knowledge and practices relative to a healthy pregnancy;
- Identifying cost-effective opportunities for the prevention of birth defects, best available care for affected children, and the support of families with a handicapped infant; and
- Recommending capacity-building, priority research, and institutional and global efforts to reduce the incidence and impact of birth defects in developing countries.[1]

---

[1]Two topics outside the scope of this report—perinatal transmission of HIV/AIDS and the effect of tobacco use during pregnancy—are discussed in the forthcoming companion report, *Improving Birth Outcomes: Meeting the Challenge in the Developing World.*

This report was developed in conjunction with a companion report, *Improving Birth Outcomes: Meeting the Challenge in the Developing World*, for which the Institute of Medicine assembled a committee with broad international expertise in fields related to birth outcomes: clinical research, epidemiology, pediatrics, neonatology, obstetrics, genetics, nutrition, and public health. The committee members were also chosen for their first-hand experience in maternal and neonatal health in a wide range of low- and middle-income countries. During the development of that report, the committee was asked to expand its work and specifically consider means of reducing the impact of birth defects in developing countries. Although most committee members give priority to the issues covered in the broader report, they recognize that several affordable interventions can have important benefits and that an increasing proportion of the overall health burden will be attributable to birth defects as countries improve infant and neonatal mortality rates. They also recognize the need for improved data on birth outcomes, including the incidence and disease burden of birth defects.

The committee had access to a large and varied body of literature from which to derive the data used for this study. These sources include bibliographic references on related topics, databases such as MEDLINE, university libraries, and the Internet sites of organizations associated with research and services for birth defects. Although much published information on these disorders in developing countries is found in international and national journals and reports, some evidence appears in local journals, proceedings of meetings, and unpublished reports prepared for the World Health Organization and other international organizations. To explore this knowledge, the committee enlisted experts with recent research experience in developing countries; these experts made workshop presentations or provided information through technical consultations.

This combination of sources, the committee believes, accurately represents the current state of knowledge regarding the epidemiology of birth defects; their prevention, treatment, and rehabilitation in developing countries; and the capacity of local health care systems to undertake similar programs. Evaluation of this evidence enabled the committee to identify gaps in knowledge and to propose operational research to improve the effectiveness and affordability of such programs. The committee's findings, strategies, and recommendations are intended to assist local ministries of health, nongovernmental organizations, and academic institutions in developing countries, as well as partner institutions, as they tailor their programs to reduce the impact of birth defects.

MAGNITUDE OF THE PROBLEM

A birth defect is any structural or functional abnormality in a neonate that is determined by factors operating before conception or during gestation. These abnormalities may be apparent immediately after birth or manifest later in life. The causes of birth defects can be grouped in three main categories: (1) *genetic* (25 to 30 percent of total birth defects), which includes chromosomal abnormalities and single-gene defects; (2) *environmental* (5 to 10 percent of total birth defects), which includes nutritional deficiencies, infectious diseases, maternal medical conditions, teratogenic medications, alcohol and recreational drugs, and teratogenic pollutants; and (3) *complex genetic and unknown* (65 to 70 percent of total birth defects), which encompasses unknown causes and probably involves more than one gene or environmental factor.

Although individually rare, birth defects taken together account for a significant proportion of morbidity and mortality among infants and children, particularly in areas where infant mortality due to more common causes has been reduced. The prevalence of specific conditions varies widely in different populations. In countries where basic public health services are not available, the birth prevalence of serious birth defects is generally higher than in developed countries. The birth defects discussed in this report were selected from the thousands of known birth defects because of their severity, their prevalence in developing countries, their representation in the medical literature from those countries, and the availability of effective prevention or treatment. At least eight conditions may contribute to a higher incidence of birth defects: (1) inadequate periconceptional intake of folic acid, (2) iodine deficiency in the mother's diet, (3) lack of vaccination against rubella, (4) women giving birth after 35 years of age, (5) consanguineous marriages, (6) alcohol consumption during pregnancy, (7) the use of teratogenic medications, and (8) the lack of prenatal diagnosis and termination of pregnancies where the fetus is severely affected.

FINDINGS AND RECOMMENDATIONS

Where resources are scarce, policy makers face difficult choices in allocating limited funds for health care. Effective strategies to address birth defects in developing countries must take into account the competing needs for resources and social, economic, and other factors that constrain health care resources. Health care systems and services vary widely both among and within countries. Thus to be effective, strategies and interventions need to be tailored to the specific population being served.

The strategy proposed in this report for significantly reducing the impact of birth defects has three stages. The first involves the introduction of highly effective and relatively inexpensive interventions to prevent birth defects. The second stage involves improving the care locally available for affected infants. The third involves genetic screening, in the form of (1) preconceptional detection of risk factors associated with birth defects; (2)

prenatal diagnosis, with termination of pregnancy offered, where legal, as an option for fetuses with confirmed severe birth defects; and (3) neonatal screening and treatment of infants with treatable genetic and metabolic diseases. The third stage has been reached in some countries in Latin America and the Middle East, where successful implementation of the most cost-effective strategies against birth defects and interventions to improve birth outcomes in general have reduced infant mortality rates to approximately 20 to 40 per 1,000 live births, and where additional resources have been available for genetic screening. At all three stages, the process of reducing birth defects involves national leadership and coordination; surveillance of birth defects and infant mortality to track progress and identify unrecognized conditions; and monitoring of interventions, even in low-resource settings, to tailor them for maximum effectiveness.

Highly Cost-Effective Interventions

Medical advances in recent decades have identified a number of affordable interventions that address the causes and risks of birth defects. Several of these have been shown to be cost-effective in developing countries. These interventions may involve public health education and campaigns; collaboration with food manufacturers, health legislators, pharmaceutical companies, and government departments responsible for environmental issues; or the expansion of established services in maternal and child health, infectious disease control, nutrition, and other primary care programs. This report describes interventions for prevention, counseling and diagnosis, treatment, and rehabilitation, all of which are aimed at reducing the impact of birth defects. For these interventions to be fully effective, however, a strong program of basic reproductive care must be available.

Recommendation 1. Basic reproductive health care services—an essential component of primary health care in all countries—should be used to reduce the impact of birth defects by providing:

- Effective family planning,
- Education for couples on avoidable risks for birth defects,
- Effective preconceptional and prenatal care and educational campaigns to stress the importance of such care, and
- Neonatal care that permits the early detection and best care locally available for management of birth defects.

Recommendations 2 to 8 propose specific interventions that can be considered by health ministries in conjunction with their own health care priorities and implemented within the national framework of public health education and basic reproductive care.

Recommendation 2. Women should be discouraged from reproducing after age 35 to minimize the risk of chromosomal birth defects such as Down syndrome.

Recommendation 3. All women of reproductive age should routinely receive 400 micrograms of synthetic folic acid per day for the reduction of neural tube defects. This is best accomplished through fortification of widely consumed staple foods. Where fortification is not feasible or is incomplete, daily supplementation programs should be provided for women before and during pregnancy.

Recommendation 4. A program of universal fortification of salt with 25–50 milligrams of iodine per kilogram of salt used for human and animal consumption should be adopted to prevent iodine deficiency disorders.

Recommendation 5. Women should be vaccinated against rubella before they reach reproductive age to prevent congenital rubella syndrome.

Recommendation 6. Education programs and public health messages should counsel women to limit or avoid alcohol consumption during pregnancy including during the early weeks.

Recommendation 7. Education programs and public health messages should educate health care providers and women of childbearing age about the importance of avoiding locally available teratogenic medications during pregnancy.

Recommendation 8. Ministries of public health, in collaboration with other government departments in developing countries, should establish regulations to reduce occupational exposure to teratogens—such as mercury and other pollutants—and create programs to raise public awareness of the health risks, including birth defects, associated with these substances.

The burden imposed by birth defects justifies widespread implementation of these cost-effective interventions. Their success will depend upon investments in personnel, training, micronutrients, vaccines, medications, and infrastructure. Variability among communities in the perception of birth defects, expectations of what medical care can and should provide, and the cost of particular interventions complicate the identification of an effective, affordable intervention. Optimal results are obtained when services reflect local benefits and costs and when community input and evaluation are used to improve programs.

Recommendation 9. Where possible, cost-effective interventions to prevent birth defects should be provided through public health campaigns and the primary health care system. The resources necessary for their success, including staff, training, and adequate supplies of nutrients, medicines, and vaccines should be provided as well.

Provision of the Best Locally Available Care

While some disorders cannot be treated at all or only at great expense, others can be partially or largely corrected with affordable therapies. Early diagnosis provides the best chance for the effective treatment of birth defects.

Recommendation 10. Children and adults with birth defects should receive the best medical care that is available in their setting, including, where possible, medication and surgery. Treatment should be undertaken as early as possible and be provided through an organized referral process.

It is recommended that each country establish clear, realistic priorities for the treatment of birth defects. This process involves balancing costs and benefits for specific neonatal therapies and surgeries against those for other health care services. It includes consideration of promising models of low-cost rehabilitation services for those with birth defects, as well as support services for their families. Effective rehabilitation services have been established in settings with very limited financial and professional resources.

Recommendation 11. Parents of children with birth defects should be guided to organizations that provide rehabilitation for the child and psychosocial support for the child and family. Education policies at the national and local levels should ensure that all children, including those with birth defects, receive appropriate schooling.

Genetic Screening to Further Reduce the Impact of Birth Defects

Once countries have implemented the basic, highly effective strategies of reproductive health care to reduce neonatal and infant mortality outlined above, further reductions can be accomplished by addressing genetic risks for birth defects.

Recommendation 12. Countries with comprehensive systems of basic reproductive health care that have lowered infant mortality rates to the range of 20 to 40 per 1,000 can further reduce infant mortality by establishing genetic screening programs. These programs should address severe, locally prevalent conditions with clear screening and diag-

nostic tests; effective, acceptable strategies for prevention or treatment; and be cost-effective. Counseling, with the goal of enabling individuals to make free and informed health care decisions, including the choice, where legal, to terminate a pregnancy in the case of a severe birth defect, should be integral to all screening and diagnostic programs.

Ongoing Needs for National Coordination, Surveillance, and Monitoring of Interventions

The impact of individual birth defects and of birth defects in the aggregate must be known if the greatest needs are to be identified and addressed. However, a review of epidemiological and burden-of-disease statistics on birth defects in developing countries reveals a substantial lack of definitive data. Much of the information has either been extrapolated from statistics for industrialized countries or derived from hospital-based studies in developing countries. In both cases, the data are thus subject to systematic underestimation.

National baseline epidemiological data to identify patterns of occurrence of birth defects can help establish priorities for interventions and may identify unusually prevalent birth defects. Follow-up data will enable countries to track trends, calculate the burden of disease associated with birth defects, and monitor the cost and effectiveness of interventions.

Recommendation 13. Collection of epidemiological data on birth defects is necessary to understand the extent of the problem and identify intervention priorities. Depending on the infant mortality rate, the capacity of the health care system, and the resources available, countries should incrementally develop the following:

- **National demographic data on neonatal and infant mortality and morbidity,**
- **Data on causes of death,**
- **Documentation of birth defects using standardized protocols for diagnosis, and**
- **Ongoing monitoring of the common birth defects in a country or region.**

National programs of basic reproductive health should set uniform standards for training and performance; collect, interpret, and act on surveillance data; and foster communication among health care providers, researchers, and policy makers. Many organizations contribute to the strengthening of health care in developing countries. However, a coordinated national effort is necessary to support comprehensive reproductive care. Internet capabilities can facilitate these functions and provide access to the information and expertise that will be needed as countries develop their own programs to address birth defects and other issues in reproductive care.

Recommendation 14. Each country should develop a strategy to reduce the impact of birth defects, a framework of activities by which this can be accomplished, and the commitment of health leaders to accomplish these goals.

National programs of basic reproductive health should collect and interpret surveillance data, set uniform standards for the training and performance of health care providers, and foster communication among health care providers, researchers, and policy makers.

Recommendation 15. Each country should strengthen its public health capacity for recognizing and implementing interventions that have proven effective in reducing the impact of birth defects. This includes monitoring and tuning interventions for clinical- and cost-effectiveness in the local setting.

CONCLUSION

Traditionally, health initiatives in developing countries have focused on the control of infectious diseases and malnutrition to reduce infant and child mortality. The next steps to reduce infant mortality and mitigate the impact of severe, lifelong disability can involve low-cost strategies to prevent severe birth defects. At minimal cost, countries can discourage women from reproducing after they reach 35 years of age, reduce the incidence of neural tube defects by fortifying a staple food with folic acid, and reduce iodine deficiency disorders by fortifying salt with iodine. A second set of proven and cost-effective interventions involves improved treatments to reduce disabilities caused by birth defects. A third set interventions, suitable for settings in which more comprehensive health services are available, infant mortality is lower, and birth defects have become a leading cause of neonatal mortality involves preconceptional and prenatal screening to prevent genetic birth defects.

To achieve these objectives, senior policy makers must recognize the enormous personal and societal consequences of birth defects and provide leadership to reduce their impact. Surveillance, by providing data on the magnitude of birth defects, can facilitate action. Surveillance data are also key for setting priorities for specific interventions. It is hoped that the recommendations in this report will contribute to renewed efforts to reduce the impact of birth defects in the developing world.

1

Introduction

Although individually rare, birth defects taken together account for a significant proportion of mortality and morbidity among infants and children in populations where infectious diseases are largely under control and nutritional deficiencies have for the most part been corrected (Jenkins, 1977). A birth defect is any structural or functional abnormality determined by factors operating largely before conception or during gestation. These abnormalities may be apparent immediately after birth, or they may manifest later in life. Birth defects result from a variety of factors, but most cannot yet be ascribed to a specific cause (Nelson and Holmes, 1989). There are three major categories of causes: (1) genetic, (2) environmental, and (3) complex genetic or unknown.

Genetic (chromosomal and single-gene) causes are estimated to account for about 25–30 percent of total birth defects. Chromosomal anomalies have been demonstrated in about 0.5 percent of newborn infants. This number may increase as modern cytogenetic techniques identify previously unrecognized chromosomal changes. An example of this is the recent use of telomeric probes, which found that 5–7 percent of mentally retarded children have a cryptic translocation that had not been recognized using traditional techniques (Knight et al., 1999).

Approximately 1 percent of all births are characterized by a mutation at a single genetic locus. Usually there are no previously affected relatives. This is the case with lethal autosomal dominant traits, which typically arise as a result of a fresh mutation in the oocyte or sperm. Not all mutant genes manifest at birth or lead to structural malformations. However, the proportion of birth defects caused by known single-gene mutations is likely to be

11

higher than for chromosomal abnormalities, based on Nelson and Holmes' (1989) survey of nearly 70,000 newborns, in which there were three times as many single-gene mutations. Many mutations are likely to remain unrecognized until a function has been established for most of the thousands of human genes.

Environmental causes are estimated to be responsible for about 5–10 percent of total birth defects (Nelson and Holmes, 1989). Environmental causes include nutritional deficiencies, maternal illnesses, infectious agents, and teratogenic drugs. Whether an exposure causes damage depends on several factors, including the actual exposure, the stage of gestation, and the individual's genetic susceptibility.

Complex genetic or unknown causes are estimated to account for 65–70 percent of all birth defects, some of which are lethal. Complex birth defects may involve a few interacting genes (oligogenic), many genes (polygenic), the environment, or an interaction between genes and environment (multifactorial). Subtle chromosomal abnormalities may have been missed, complex genetic mechanisms may be identified when the functions of more genes are identified, and there may be previously undetected environmental influences.

Families with an affected child have an increased incidence of almost all the birth defects that are restricted to a single organ system, such as cleft lip and/or cleft palate, developmental hip dysplasia, and most forms of cardiac anomalies (Simpson and Golbus, 1992). After the birth of an affected child, the risk that a subsequent child will be affected is typically 2–5 percent, which is many times higher than the incidence in the general population (less than 0.1 per cent for most single-organ malformations), but lower than the 25–50 percent expected if the etiology were due to a single gene.

The birth defects discussed in this report (see Table 1-1) were selected from the thousands of known birth defects because of their severity, their prevalence in developing countries, and their representation in the medical literature from these countries. What is known, and not known, about these selected birth defects—their prevalence, burden of disease, biological origins, associated risk factors, prevention, and treatment—serve as the evidence base for the recommendations presented in this report on reducing the impact of birth defects in developing countries.

MAGNITUDE OF THE PROBLEM

The prevalence of specific birth defects varies widely with the ethnic, geographic, cultural, and economic characteristics of populations (Kuliev and Modell, 1990). The combined prevalence of all birth defects is estimated to be about 4–5 percent of live births in developed countries (Kuliev and Modell, 1990; World Health Organization, 1999; Penchaszadeh, 1994).

TABLE 1-1 Causes, Classification, and Examples of Selected Birth Defects[a]

Cause	Classification	Birth Defect Examples
Genetic	Chromosomal	Down syndrome Trisomy 18 Trisomy 13
	Single gene	α- and β-Thalassemias Sickle cell disorder G6PD[b] deficiency Oculocutaneous albinism Cystic fibrosis Phenylketonuria Hemophilia A and B
Environmental (teratogenic)	Infectious diseases	Congenital rubella syndrome Congenital cytomegalovirus Toxoplasmosis
	Other maternal illness	Insulin-dependent diabetes mellitus Phenylketonuria Hyperthermia

	Maternal nutritional deficiencies
	  Folic acid
	  Iodine
		
		Neural tube defects
		Iodine deficiency disorders

	Medications
	  Thalidomide
	  Misoprostol
	  Anticonvulsants
	  Anticoagulants
		
		Reduction deformities of limbs
		Several
		Several
		Neurological damage

	Recreational drugs Alcohol	 Fetal alcohol syndrome
	Pollutants Organic mercury	 Neurological damage
	Ionizing radiation	Neurological damage
Complex genetic and unknown	Congenital malformations involving single organ systems	Congenital heart disease Neural tube defects Cleft lip and/or cleft palate Talipes or clubfoot Developmental dysplasia of the hip

[a]These birth defects were selected on the basis of severity, prevalence in developing countries, and representation in the medical literature of developing countries.
[b]G6PD = glucose-6-phosphate dehydrogenase.

In the developing countries with stronger health care systems and more complete data on birth defects, the birth prevalence of recognizable birth defects is estimated to be similar to that in developed countries (about 2–3 percent) (Castilla and Lopez-Camelo, 1990; International Clearinghouse for Birth Defects Monitoring Systems, 1998; Heredero, 1992; Delport et al., 1995; Venter et al., 1995; World Health Organization, 1997). Rates may be higher in some developing countries, underscoring the need for better surveillance data. Prevalence at birth represents only part of the total prevalence of birth defects because many conditions are not recognized for months or years after birth (Christianson et al., 1981; World Health Organization, 1997; Venter et al., 1995).

Global burden-of-disease data from 1990 show congenital anomalies to be the tenth leading cause of disability-adjusted life years in developing countries. This estimate, although the best available, is limited by a lack of accurate data on birth defects in many countries and by inadequate data on infants and children for conditions not detected at birth (Murray and Lopez, 1997; World Health Organization, 1999, 2000). What is certain, however, is that birth defects have a severe impact on individuals and their families because they manifest early in development and can cause early death or lifelong impairment. The prognosis for many children with birth defects can be improved only through surgical procedures, which may not be available or affordable. Even those who receive treatment may require long-term care from their families—a particular hardship for families in which more than one member is affected (Penchaszadeh, 1994). Birth defects therefore diminish the productivity and quality of life for affected individuals, for their families and communities, and ultimately for society as a whole.

INCREASE IN THE IMPORTANCE OF BIRTH DEFECTS WITH DECREASING INFANT MORTALITY

Over the last four decades, the average infant mortality rate in developing countries has fallen from 137 to 66 per 1000 live births, largely as a result of improvements in safe childbirth and control of infectious diseases and malnutrition. Progress in lowering infant mortality rates has, however, varied greatly among developing countries. Those that have made the least progress toward this goal—located mainly in sub-Saharan Africa and South Asia—tend to have weaker health care systems (United Nations Children's Fund, 1998). Early progress in sub-Saharan Africa has been checked by the HIV/AIDS epidemic.[1] Most perinatal deaths in sub-Saharan Africa and

---

[1]Although further discussion of HIV/AIDS is beyond the scope of this report, perinatal transmission of HIV/AIDS is discussed in detail in a companion report, *Improving Birth Outcomes: Meeting the Challenge in the DevelopingWorld*, also authored by this committee.

South Asia are caused by complicated deliveries, birth asphyxia, infections, and low birth weight. In these settings, infant mortality is best addressed by focusing on cost-effective medical services for basic reproductive care and safe delivery, control of infectious diseases, and treatment of nutritional inadequacies (Jenkins, 1977; Stoll and Measham, 2001).

The most impressive reductions in infant mortality rates over the last four decades have been in Latin America and the Caribbean (from 105 to 35 per 1,000 live births), East Asia and the Pacific (133 to 41 per 1,000), and the Middle East and North Africa (154 to 50 per 1,000) (United Nations Children's Fund, 1998). By 1997, infant mortality rates had declined to less than 40 per 1,000 live births in 67 of the 142 developing countries, and 8 more countries had rates between 41 and 50 per 1,000. The population of the 75 countries with infant mortality rates below 50 per 1,000 was 2.8 billion, which represents 60 percent of the population of the developing world (United Nations Children's Fund, 1998).

As infant mortality rates fall, birth defects are responsible for an increasing proportion of the infant mortality and morbidity (Modell and Kuliev, 1989; World Health Organization, 1997, 1999). In the majority of Latin American and Middle Eastern countries that have reduced infant mortality to less than 50 per 1,000, the infant mortality due to birth defects is as high as 25 percent (World Health Organization, 1997), which is similar to the proportion in developed countries.

The increasing role of birth defects in countries that have lowered infant mortality rates is reflected in admissions to pediatric hospitals: 8–19 percent of total admissions in Middle Eastern Countries (World Health Organization, 1997) and 10–25 percent in some urban centers in Latin America. These hospital stays also tend to be longer and more expensive (Penchaszadeh, 1979; Carnevale et al., 1985).

REDUCING BIRTH DEFECTS IN COUNTRIES
WITH LOW INFANT MORTALITY

Figure 1-1 shows decreases in the infant mortality rate over the last two decades for North Africa, the Middle East, and Pakistan. As these rates have decreased to a range of 20 to 40 per 1,000, several countries in these regions have introduced genetic screening programs for specific birth defects (Alwan and Modell, 1997). Such programs are less cost-effective than interventions that address basic reproductive care, but they have been identified by these countries as the next essential step in lowering infant mortality rates cost-effectively. In 1981, Cuba established national genetic screening in primary care programs, with referral to secondary and tertiary health care (Heredero, 1992). Cyprus, South Africa, and Iran also have primary care programs with genetic screening for specific birth defects (see Boxes 3-

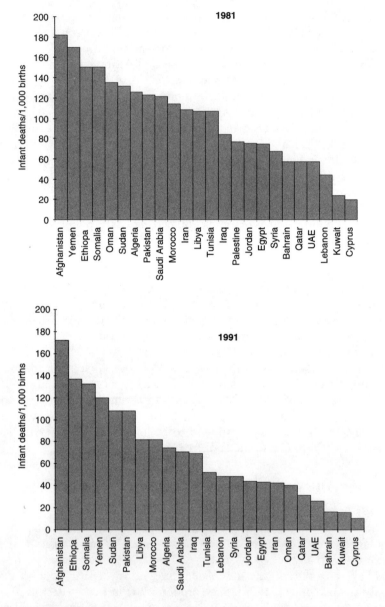

FIGURE 1-1 Infant mortality rates in North Africa, the Middle East, and Pakistan over two decades.

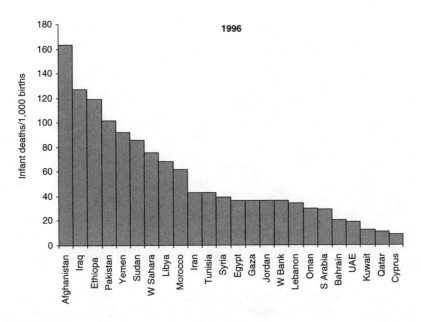

FIGURE 1-1 continued
SOURCE: Alwin and Modell, 1997.

1 and 3-6 in Chapter 3) (Christianson et al., 1995; Christianson, 2000; Gaudet, 1999; Khoury et al., 2000). In many other developing countries, including India and several in Latin America, genetic screening services are accessible only to middle- and high-income patients in the tertiary care centers of major cities (Jenkins, 1990; Penchaszadeh, 1992, 1993).

SOCIAL, ECONOMIC, AND HEALTH CONTEXT

Effective strategies to address birth defects in developing countries must consider the competing health needs of these populations, as well as a variety of social, economic, and health system–specific factors that limit resources for health care. These factors include the following (World Health Organization, 1999):

• Financial resources: The average per capita gross national products of developing countries are 10 to 40 times lower than those of developed countries.
• Income distribution: Extreme income inequalities result in a smaller proportion of the population having access to quality health care. In fact,

about one-quarter of the combined population of all developing countries survives on less than $1 per day.

• Education: Literacy rates in developing countries range from 57 to 87 percent and are generally lower among women than men.

• Fertility: Developing-country fertility rates are high relative to those of developed countries, particularly among less-educated women.

• Infrastructure: Developing-country populations frequently lack access to safe water (70 percent), adequate sanitation (42 percent), transportation, and communication.

• Infant mortality: Rates of infant mortality in the developing world vary—from as low as 9 deaths per 1,000 live births in Cuba to as high as 191 per 1,000 live births in Niger.

• Burden of disease: By the end of the twentieth century, about 42 percent of all deaths in developing countries were caused by avoidable conditions such as infectious diseases, lack of reproductive health care, and nutritional deficiencies, compared with 6 percent in developed countries.

To address these challenges, programs must be tailored to the needs and resources of communities in each country. The recommendations in this report are intended to guide the development of a capacity to address birth defects that is integrated with and builds on current health care services for mothers, infants, and children.

STUDY PURPOSE

Despite major improvements in the knowledge of birth defects, their incidence and impact remain high in most countries. As infant and neonatal mortality decline, an increasing proportion of adverse outcomes at birth are due to birth defects. This study addresses the steps needed to improve the prevention of and care for birth defects by:

• Reviewing current knowledge and practices for a healthy pregnancy;
• Identifying cost-effective opportunities for prevention of birth defects and support of families with a handicapped infant; and
• Recommending capacity-building, priority research, and institutional and global efforts to reduce the incidence and impact of birth defects in developing countries.

This report is intended to engage a broad spectrum of individuals and organizations that have the potential to lead efforts to address the global impact of birth defects. Such individuals and groups include, but are not limited to, policy makers, health ministries, United Nations agencies, multilateral development banks, international donor agencies, foundations, nongovernmental organizations, professional societies, pharmaceutical and medical-device companies, advocacy groups, health care professionals, researchers, consumer and patient advocacy groups, and interested members of the public. This diverse and influential audience holds the key to raising public awareness and generating the commitment and resources necessary to reduce the burden of birth defects in developing countries.

STUDY APPROACH

The Institute of Medicine (IOM) assembled a study committee with broad international expertise in public health, neonatology, obstetrics, genetics, epidemiology, pediatrics, and clinical research to prepare a report on improving birth outcomes in developing countries. The committee members are listed at the beginning of the report (biographies are provided in Appendix B). This report was prepared by the committee with the assistance of expert consultants to more fully address the issues involved in reducing birth defects. Although most committee members give highest priority to the issues covered in the broader report, they acknowledge the lack of epidemiological information on the rates and disease burden of birth defects in many developing countries; the potential value of several affordable interventions; and, as countries reduce neonatal and infant mortality rates, the increasing proportion of the disease burden caused by birth defects.

The data used for this study were assembled from bibliographic references on related topics and from databases such as MEDLINE, university libraries, and Internet sites of organizations associated with research and services for birth defects. Although much of the published information on these disorders in developing countries was found in international and national journals and reports, some of the evidence has appeared in local journals, proceedings of meetings, and unpublished reports prepared for the World Health Organization and other international organizations. To tap this broad knowledge base, the committee enlisted experts with recent research or service experience in developing countries. Data and evidence were provided by these experts through workshop presentations and technical consultation on the report chapters. The framework for the committee's examination of birth defects included an overview of epidemiological parameters; review of the current knowledge base on interventions; and examination of the feasibility, cost, and impact of proposed interventions. This combination of evidence, the committee believes, is an accurate representation of the state of knowledge concerning the epidemiology of birth defects, their prevention and care in developing countries, and the capacity of local health care systems to undertake prevention and care programs. Evaluation of this evidence enabled the committee to identify gaps in knowledge and to propose strategies for operational research to fill these gaps.

ORGANIZATION OF THE REPORT

The next three chapters address the challenges of birth defects in developing countries. Chapter 2 describes the causes of the major classes and types of birth defects, epidemiological parameters, and the burden of disease in low-resource settings. Chapter 3 describes interventions that can reduce the impact of birth defects: first those that are effective and affordable in settings with limited resources, and then screening services for genetic birth defects that are appropriate for countries in which infant and neonatal mortality rates have been lowered using the most cost-effective interventions. Examples of interventions from developing countries are described in boxes throughout the text. Chapter 4 provides a framework for implementing such interventions in primary health care systems.

REFERENCES

Alwan AA, Modell B. 1997. Community control of genetic and congenital disorders. Technical publication series, No 24. Alexandria, Egypt. World Health Organization Regional Office for the Eastern Mediterranean.

Carnevale A, Hernandez M, Reyes R, Paz F, Sosa C. 1985. The frequency and economic burden of genetic disease in a pediatric hospital in Mexico City. *American Journal of Medical Genetics* 20(4):665–675.

Castilla EE, Lopez-Camelo JS. 1990. The surveillance of birth defects in South America: I. The search for time clusters: Epidemics. *Advances in Mutagenesis Research* 2:191–210.

Christianson AL. 2000. Medical genetics in primary health care. *Indian Journal of Pediatrics* 67(11):831–835.

Christianson AL, Gericke GS, Venter PA, du Toit JL. 1995. Genetics, primary health care and the Third World. *South African Medical Journal* 85(1):6–7.

Christianson RE, van den Berg BJ, Milkovich L, Oechsli FW. 1981. Incidence of congenital anomalies among white and black live births with long-term follow-up. *American Journal of Public Health* 71(12):1333–1341.

Delport SD, Christianson AL, van den Berg HJ, Wolmarans L, Gericke GS. 1995. Congenital anomalies in black South African liveborn neonates at an urban academic hospital. *South African Medical Journal* 85(1):11–15.

Gaudet D. 1999. From DNA to the community. *Community Genetics* 2(4):139–140.

Heredero L. 1992. Comprehensive national genetic program in a developing country—Cuba. *Birth Defects Original Article Series* 28(3):52–57.

International Clearinghouse for Birth Defects Monitoring Systems (ICBDMS). 1998. *World Atlas of Birth Defects*. 1st edition. ICBD and European Register of Congenital Abnormalities and Twins (EUROCAT).

Jenkins T. 1977. The role of screening in the prevention of inherited disease in South Africa. *South African Medical Journal* 51(23):832–837.

Jenkins T. 1990. Medical genetics in South Africa. *Journal of Medical Genetics* 27(12):760–779.

Khoury MJ, Burke W, Thomson EJ (eds.). 2000. *Genetics and Public Health in the 21st Century: Using Genetic Information to Improve Health and Prevent Disease*. New York: Oxford University Press.

Knight SJL, Regan R, Nicod A, Horsley SW, Kearney L, Homfray T. 1999. Subtle chromosomal rearrangements in children with unexplained mental retardation. *Lancet* 354(9191):1676–1681.

Kuliev A, Modell B. 1990. Problems in the control of genetic disorders. *Biomedical Science* 1(1):3–17.

Modell B, Kuliev AM. 1989. Impact of public health on human genetics. *Clinical Genetics* 36(5):286–298.

Murray CJ, Lopez AD. 1997. Regional patterns of disability-free life expectancy and disability-adjusted life expectancy: Global Burden of Disease Study. *Lancet* 349(9062):1347–1352.

Nelson K, Holmes LB. 1989. Malformations due to presumed spontaneous mutations in newborn infants. *New England Journal of Medicine* 320(1):19–23.

Penchaszadeh VB. 1979. Frequency and characteristics of birth defects admissions to a pediatric hospital in Venezuela. *American Journal of Medical Genetics* 3(4):359–369.

Penchaszadeh VB. 1992. Implementing comprehensive genetic services in developing countries: Latin America. *Birth Defects Original Article Series* 28(3):17–26.

Penchaszadeh VB. 1993. Reproductive health and genetic testing in the Third World. *Clinical Obstetrics and Gynecology* 36(3):485–495.

Penchaszadeh VB. 1994. Genetics and public health. *Bulletin of the Pan American Health Organization* 28(1):62–72.

Simpson and Golbus, 1992. *Genetics in Obstetrics and Gynecology.* 2nd edition. Philadelphia: W.B. Saunders.

Stoll BJ, Measham AR. 2001. Children can't wait: Improving the future for the world's poorest infants. *Journal of Pediatrics* 139(5):729–733.

United Nations Children's Fund (UNICEF). 1998. *The State of the World's Children 1999.* New York: UNICEF.

United Nations Children's Fund (UNICEF). 2000. *The State of the World's Children 2001.* New York: UNICEF.

Venter PA, Christianson AL, Hutamo CM, Makhura MP, Gericke GS. 1995. Congenital anomalies in rural black South African neonates—a silent epidemic? *South African Medical Journal* 85(1):15–20.

World Health Organization (WHO). 1997. Alwan AA, Modell B (eds.). *Community Control of Genetic and Congenital Disorders.* Alexandria, Egypt: WHO.

World Health Organization (WHO). 1999. *Human Genetics: Services for the Prevention and Management of Genetic Disorders and Birth Defects in Developing Countries: Report of a Joint WHO/WOAPBD Meeting.* Geneva: WHO.

World Health Organization (WHO). 2000. *Primary Health Care Approaches for the Prevention and Control of Congenital Genetic Disorders: Report of a WHO Meeting.* Geneva: WHO.

2

Impact and Patterns of Occurrence

irth defects are, in the aggregate, a significant health problem for infants worldwide. The prevalence of individual conditions in different populations varies with the health care system; use and coverage of preventive strategies; and access to prenatal screening, diagnosis, and possible termination of pregnancy for severe birth defects (Kuliev and Modell, 1990; World Health Organization, 1997, 1999). Data on birth defects in several countries are given in Appendix A (Table A-1). At birth the prevalence is generally in the range of 10–60 per 1,000 live births depending on the conditions included. This number increases when assessments are made at one or five years.

To understand the patterns of occurrence of birth defects, a system for collecting and monitoring reliable data is needed. Many developing countries lack health-related statistics and registries, and about one-third of all births in these countries—an estimated 40 million each year—are not registered (Murray and Lopez, 1996; World Health Organization, 1997, 1999; United Nation Children's Fund, 1998). Thus in much of the world, it is difficult to calculate the birth prevalence of birth defects with any precision because the number of infants afflicted and the total number of surviving infants born within a specified time period is not measured. In these circumstances, birth rates and the birth prevalence of disease are approximated from hospital- and community-based studies, which are not necessarily representative of the population as a whole or even the broader community.

Notwithstanding these limitations, several studies have established that birth defects are a public health problem in developing countries. In addition, some large-scale programs monitor the occurrence of birth defects in specific regions of the world. These include the International Clearinghouse for Birth Defects Monitoring System (ICBDMS) (see Box 2-1); the Latin American Collaborative Study of Congenital Malformations (ECLAMC) (see Box 2-2); the Chinese Birth Defects Monitoring Program (CBDMP); and the European Register of Congenital Abnormalities and Twins (EURO-CAT), a network of 20 regional registries. Data from these programs and from the research literature inform this chapter's descriptions of the pathology of birth defects and their patterns of occurrence in developing countries. In this chapter and the next, three categories of causes of birth defects are discussed: genetic, environmental, and complex genetic and unknown (defined in Chapter 1).

GENETIC BIRTH DEFECTS

Of the birth defects for which a cause has been established, most are due to chromosomal disorders and single-gene mutations.

Chromosomal Disorders

Sporadic (nonhereditary) losses or rearrangements of genetic material affect at least 10 percent of conceptions, 90 percent of which end in spontaneous abortion. Surviving infants may have a congenital malformation, mental retardation, and/or disorders in sexual differentiation (World Health Organization, 1999). Data from the United States, Canada, and Germany show a birth prevalence of chromosomal abnormalities of 5 per 1,000 live

---

**BOX 2-1   International Clearinghouse for
Birth Defects Monitoring Systems**

The ICBDMS was established in 1974 to promote the exchange of information among member programs that monitor trends in the prevalence of birth defects. It monitors approximately 3 million births annually in 24 countries. ICBDMS assists local registries of congenital malformation in the identification and prevention of birth defects, so that they may serve as early warning systems to avoid the spread of epidemics of congenital malformations. The agency also promotes the exchange of information on the occurrence of birth defects in populations; consults in investigations of changes in the occurrence of birth defects; and provides training in the monitoring and epidemiology of birth defects. The *World Atlas of Birth Defects*, created by the ICBDMS in collaboration with the World Health Organization and EUROCAT, presents data from birth defects registries throughout the world.

SOURCE: World Atlas of Birth Defects, 2001.

**BOX 2-2   ECLAMC: A Clinical–Epidemiological
Research Program in Latin America**

ECLAMC, initiated in Argentina in 1967, is one of the few systems for monitoring the birth prevalence of birth defects in developing countries. Accurate, comprehensive data on most countries are sparse. Since 1974 more than 5 million neonates have been examined in selected maternity hospitals in South American countries. Of these, 100,000 neonates with birth defects have been recorded, along with an equal number of matched controls.

Various methods are used to ensure that clinical diagnoses are accurate. Difficult cases are referred to a clinical review committee, based in Rio de Janeiro, which examines photographs and other descriptive data, such as family histories. If the committee is unable to concur on a diagnosis, the data are placed on a private Web site for evaluation by a larger body of clinical geneticists in the ECLAMC network. ECLAMC dysmorphologists meet annually to discuss individual cases and train physicians in participating hospitals.

ECLAMC also uses its baseline epidemiological data to monitor and support the prevention of birth defects; systematically evaluates information concerning increased rates of a given birth defect or exposure to a given potential teratogen; identifies geographic clusters of birth defects; provides information on the prevalence and risk factors associated with several specific types of birth defects; and maintains a DNA and cell bank of selected birth defects.

SOURCE: ECLAMC, 2001; Castilla and Lopez-Camelo, 1990.

---

births (Hook, 1982); however, the birth prevalence may be higher in populations in which women continue to have children after age 35. This occurs more commonly in countries that lack family planning and access to contraceptives (World Health Organization, 1999). As Table 2-1 shows, the risk of chromosomal abnormalities, and of Down syndrome in particular, increases rapidly with advancing maternal age (Hook, 1981).

Chromosomal nondisjunction—an error in cell division that admits three, rather than two, copies of one of the chromosome 21 into the cells of the affected zygote—causes Down syndrome, in which three copies (trisomy) of chromosome 21 are present. Trisomies of chromosomes 13 and 18 are also relatively common in live-born infants. Advanced maternal age is the only well-documented risk factor for nondisjunction; however, the mechanism behind the age effect is not well understood (Nicolaidis and Petersen, 1998). Young maternal age (Croen and Shaw, 1995) and advanced paternal age (Kuliev and Modell, 1990) have also been associated with increased risk for birth defects in some, but not all, developed countries. Maternal age-adjusted risks for chromosomal numerical anomalies show little variation across racial and ethnic groups (Carothers et al., 2001).

TABLE 2-1   Maternal Age and Chromosome Abnormalities in Liveborns

Maternal Age	Risk for Down Syndrome	Total Risk for Chromosomal Abnormalities
20	1/1,667	1/526
21	1/1,667	1/526
22	1/1,429	1/500
23	1/1,429	1/500
24	1/1,250	1/476
25	1/1,250	1/476
26	1/1,176	1/476
27	1/1,111	1/455
28	1/1,053	1/435
29	1/1,000	1/417
30	1/952	1/417
31	1/909	1/385
32	1/769	1/322
33	1/602	1/286
34	1/485	1/238
35	1/378	1/192
36	1/289	1/156
37	1/224	1/127
38	1/173	1/102
39	1/136	1/83
40	1/106	1/66
41	1/82	1/53
42	1/63	1/42
43	1/49	1/33
44	1/38	1/26
45	1/30	1/21
46	1/23	1/16
47	1/18	1/13
48	1/14	1/10
49	1/11	1/8

SOURCE: Hook, 1981.

Down syndrome (Trisomy 21)

This is a common chromosomal disorder in which a child is born with three—not two—copies of chromosome 21. It causes varying degrees of mental and growth retardation, a characteristic facial appearance, and multiple malformations. It is associated with a major risk for heart malformations, a risk of duodenal atresia in which part of the small intestine is not developed, and a small but significant risk of acute leukemia. It frequently results in spontaneous abortion. Congenital heart disease associated with Down syndrome can be fatal and is the major cause of death. Inadequate intellectual development can cause severe, lifelong disability and dependence.

The estimated birth prevalence of Down syndrome in developing countries is higher than in developed countries (see Appendix A, Table A-2) (Kuliev and Modell, 1990; World Health Organization, 1996). The higher prevalence parallels the greater proportion of births to women over 35 years of age noted above—an average of 11–15 percent in developing countries versus 5–9 percent in most developed countries. The rates in Catholic countries, such as Ireland and Italy, are closer to those in developing countries. For example, the higher birth prevalence of Down syndrome in South America (1.5/1,000), compared with the average in developed countries (1/1,000), can be explained by the higher mean maternal age in that region (Castilla and Lopez-Camelo, 1990).

Early infant and childhood mortality from congenital heart disease and other conditions associated with Down syndrome result in a low population prevalence of the syndrome in most developing countries (Zhang et al., 1991). In South Africa, three-quarters of children with Down syndrome die before reaching 2 years of age (Christianson, 1996). In South America, 34 percent of Down syndrome infants with congenital heart disease—and 21 percent without heart problems—die before the age of 1 year, about twice the rate in the United Kingdom (Castilla et al., 1998).

Trisomy 18

Children with this syndrome have three instead of two copies of chromosome 18. The condition causes multiple malformations, profound mental retardation, and usually death in the first few months. It occurs in about 1 per 8,000 live births (Hook, 1992) and among stillborn infants. About three times as many females as males are born with trisomy 18, but the ratios are more equal among stillborns and spontaneously aborted fetuses.

Trisomy 13

Children with this syndrome have three instead of two copies of chromosome 13. They have multiple malformations, profound mental retardation, and generally die soon after birth or in infancy. The condition occurs in 1 in 20,000 live-born infants (Hook, 1992) and is frequently observed in spontaneously aborted fetuses. This trisomy results in pronounced retardation of intrauterine and postnatal growth and development. Nearly 50 percent of affected newborns die in their first month, and fewer than 5 percent survive past 3 years of age (Magenis et al., 1968).

Single-Gene Disorders

More than 6,000 single-gene (Mendelian or monogenic) disorders have been described (World Health Organization, 1997; Online Mendelian Inheritance in Man, 2002), and many more are suspected. These disorders are individually rare but, taken together, are estimated to account for a global birth prevalence of 10 per 1,000 live births (World Health Organization, 1999). Single-gene disorders are classified by mode of inheritance as autosomal recessive or dominant or as X-linked recessive or dominant. For autosomal recessive traits to be expressed, two copies of the mutated gene must be present; thus, if both parents are carriers of the same disease-causing recessive gene, each child has a 25 percent chance of having the disease.

Pregnancies from consanguineous marriages—marriages generally of first cousins and including second cousins—have an increased birth prevalence of autosomal recessive diseases, which increases the risk of stillbirth, neonatal and childhood death, mental retardation, and birth defects compared with pregnancies among unrelated couples (Jaber et al., 1992). In most Western urban populations, the frequency of consanguineous marriages (Castilla et al., 1991) and of births produced from these marriages (Liascovich et al., 2001) is between 1 per 1,000 and 1 per 100. In areas where consanguineous marriage is intrinsic to the culture, including parts of the Middle East, South Asia, and Africa (Bittles et al., 1991; Khlat and Khoury, 1991; Khlat et al., 1997; Durkin et al., 1998; Mokhtar et al., 1998), 20–60 percent of all marriages involve consanguineous unions. Worldwide, consanguineous marriages occur regularly in at least 20 percent of the population, and as many as 8 percent of all children worldwide have parents who are related (Kuliev and Modell, 1990; World Health Organization, 1996; Hussain and Bittles, 1998; Christianson et al., 2000).

The relationship between consanguinity and birth defects has been explored in several studies. In one study, for example, 93 percent of Palestinian Arabs who are parents of children with rare autosomal disorders were found to be related, compared with a consanguinity rate of 44 percent among the general population (Zlotogora, 1997). This study also found higher-than-average rates of consanguinity among parents of children with neural tube defects (NTDs), cleft lip and palate, and other congenital malformations. NTDs were shown to be associated with consanguinity in studies conducted in the United Arab Emirates (Al-Gazali et al., 1999) and in Saudi Arabia (Murshid, 2000). Major malformations (including but not limited to nervous system anomalies) were found at significantly higher rates among children of consanguineous parents in south India (Kulkarni and Kurian, 1990) and in an Israeli Arab community (Jaber et al., 1992).

The single-gene disorders best documented in developing countries include hemoglobin disorders, such as thalassemia and sickle cell disease, and glucose-6-phosphate dehydrogenase deficiency; oculocutaneous albinism, important in Africa; cystic fibrosis, the most common potentially fatal genetic disease among Caucasians, long considered rare in non-Caucasian populations but recently attracting increased attention; phenylketonuria (PKU); and hemophilia A and B. For several hemoglobinopathies, including α- and β-thalassemia and sickle cell disease, the mutation that causes the disorder also interferes with infection by the malaria parasite. This confers a selective advantage on carriers living in malaria-endemic areas, thereby explaining the increased frequency of these hemoglobinopathies in populations of African and Mediterranean ancestry.

Thalassemias

These are a group of inherited blood disorders in which production of hemoglobin is deficient as a result of mutations in the genes that synthesize the α- and β-globin chains of the hemoglobin. Abnormal hemoglobin (Hb) genes are believed to have originated in Africa, Asia, and the Mediterranean basin and may have remained at high frequencies because of the previously noted selective advantage of malaria resistance conferred on the heterozygous carriers of such genes, who do not usually exhibit symptoms of thalassemia (Weatherall, 1997; Sweeting et al., 1998). Thalassemias are generally more prevalent than sickle cell disorders in the Eastern Mediterranean region, North Africa, South Asia, East Asia, and the Pacific.

β-Thalassemia, the most common thalassemia, involves a defect in the production of β-globin chains, which decreases production of normal adult hemoglobin (Hb A). It occurs most often among people of Mediterranean descent. Clinically this condition includes β-thalassemia major, the homozygous state, and β-thalassemia minor, the heterozygous (carrier) state, which is usually asymptomatic. Children with β-thalassemia major do not present symptoms in the first months of life, then, in the second 6 months, they often fail to thrive and may suffer from recurrent bacterial infections, severe anemia, hepatosplenomegaly, and bone expansion, which give rise to classical thalassemia facies. Left untreated, severe β-thalassemia is fatal in childhood or early adolescence; with regular transfusions, patients live into their twenties and even longer if treated to prevent iron overload. Because of the difficulty and expense of treatment, children with β-thalassemia in poorer countries rarely receive adequate care and die young (Weatherall and Clegg, 2001).

α-Thalassemia, the heterozygous state (with a single gene for α-thalassemia) is innocuous or harmless. The homozygous state (with both genes for α-thalassemia) can be lethal before birth. The compound heterozygous forms produce a condition of variable severity known as Hb H disease, with symptoms that include moderate to severe (transfusion-dependent) anemia and splenomegaly. α-Thalassemia is most prevalent in Asia.

Several populations have been screened to determine the prevalence of thalassemia genes and traits (see Appendix A, Table A-3); α and β-thalassemia have a high incidence in a broad geographical band extending across the Mediterranean basin and parts of Africa, through the Middle East, and across India, Southeast Asia, and the Pacific Islands (see Figure 2-1). In these areas, carrier frequency for β-thalassemia ranges from 1 to 20 percent. Carriers of the milder form of β-thalassemia range from 10 to 20 percent of the population in parts of sub-Saharan Africa to 40 percent or more in parts of the Middle East and India, and higher in northern Papua New Guinea. Carriers of the more severe form of α-thalassemia occur at

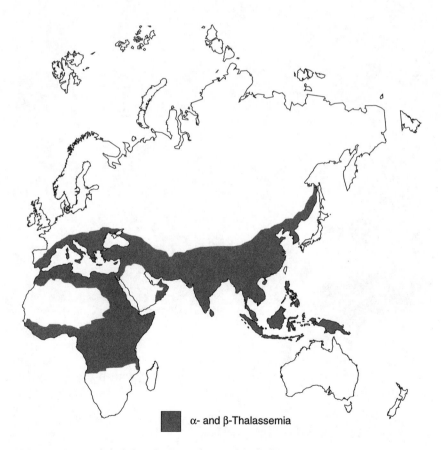

α- and β-Thalassemia

FIGURE 2-1 Global distribution of α- and β-thalassemia.
SOURCE: World Health Organization, 2001.

high frequencies only in parts of Southeast Asia and the Mediterranean basin; therefore, α-thalassemias pose less of a global health problem than β-thalassemias (Weatherall and Clegg, 2001).

Sickle cell disease

This is a genetic blood disease that results from the pairing of an abnormal hemoglobin S (HbS) with another abnormal hemoglobin. Heterozygote carriers have the largely asymptomatic sickle cell trait (HbAS); homozygotes (HbSS) have variable symptoms and are said to have sickle cell anemia; and HbS compound heterozygotes, the most prevalent being

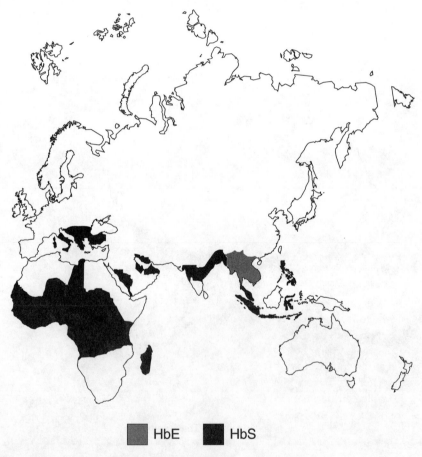

HbE   HbS

FIGURE 2-2 Global distribution of hemoglobins S and E.
SOURCE: World Health Organization, 2001.

hemoglobin C (HbSC) and hemoglobin E (HbSE), have the most severe symptoms. The global distribution of hemoglobins S and E is shown in Figure 2-2. The hemoglobin molecules in red blood cells stick to one another and cause the red cells to become crescent or sickle shaped. Sickled cells cannot pass easily through tiny blood vessels.

Sickle cell disease affects millions of people worldwide but is particularly common among people from sub-Saharan Africa; Spanish-speaking regions; Saudi Arabia; India; and Mediterranean countries. The high frequency of sickle cell disease in these populations is attributed to the lower rates of mortality from malaria infection among carriers, who are asymptomatic, compared with noncarriers (Ashley-Koch et al., 2000). Relatively high rates of consanguineous marriage in the Eastern Mediterranean region have increased the prevalence of sickle cell disease in that population as well (World Health Organization, 1997).

Children with homozygous sickle cell disease or sickle cell anemia are susceptible to episodes of painful vaso-occlusive crises and chronic anemia and are at increased risk for developing infections, particularly *Streptococcus pneumoniae*, which can cause fatal sepsis, meningitis, or pneumonia. In sub-Saharan Africa, many children with sickle cell anemia die early in life (Weatherall and Clegg, 2001). While survival is influenced by several variables, there is a general correlation with the frequency of crises. Extensive vaso-occlusive crises can cause ischemic damage and infarction, with resulting splenic dysfunction, "acute chest syndrome," impaired renal function, and stroke. Patients with more than three crises per year live to a median age of 35 years, while those with fewer than one per year may live into their forties (Fauci et al., 2001).

Epidemiological studies of sickle cell disease have reported a wide range of prevalence rates among, and even within, developing countries (see Appendix A, Table A-4). In Nigeria, sickle cell carrier frequencies have been estimated at 25 percent in the south and 19–33 percent in the north (Akinyanju, 1989). HbC is less common in this population, but carrier rates of 5–7 percent have been reported in the Yoruba of southwest Nigeria. Combined, these carrier rates would be expected to result in about 90,000 births per year in Nigeria alone. However, the prevalence of the disease in the general population is low because 70 percent of patients with sickle cell anemia (HbSS) die undiagnosed in childhood (Akinyanju, 1989; Angastiniotis et al., 1995).

Sickle cell disease is also common in countries with a high proportion of African migrants. Thus in Cuba, where 30–40 percent of the population has African ancestry, the carrier frequency is 3–6 percent (Granda et al., 1991, 1994); in Brazil, the carrier frequency among people of mixed ancestry is 4.7 percent and among people of African origin is 6.2 percent (Salzano, 1985).

Glucose-6-phosphate dehydrogenase (G6PD) deficiency

This enzyme defect results from recessive mutations in the gene for the enzyme G6PD, which is carried on the X chromosome. Hundreds of variants of G6PD deficiency have been identified among the 400 million people estimated to be affected worldwide. Individuals deficient in G6PD are vulnerable to developing acute hemolytic anemia as a result of infections, exposure to oxidant drugs (the antimalarial, primaquine, and the sulfonamide antibiotics or sulfones), or chemicals (naphthalene in mothballs), or ingestion of fava beans. Severe hemolysis in these cases can be fatal (Steensma et al., 2001). Some affected newborns develop severe hemolytic jaundice and kernicterus, which can result in death or serious neurologic impairment.

The disorder is most prevalent in Central, West, and East Africa; the Eastern Mediterranean; and South and East Asia (Verjee, 1993; El-Hazmi and Warsy, 1996; World Health Organization, 1989, 1996, 1997). As with thalassemias and sickle cell disease, carriers of G6PD deficiency have a selective advantage against infection by malaria (Roth et al., 1983), which increases the frequency of these carriers in populations of African and Mediterranean ancestries (Allison and Clyde, 1961).

About 7.5 percent of the world's population carry a gene for G6PD deficiency, and about 3 percent are deficient in the enzyme; however, there is large regional variability. In Africa, for example, carrier frequencies as high as 35 percent have been reported (World Health Organization, 1989). Appendix A (Table A-5) lists selected studies of G6PD prevalence among groups ranging from children in a few schools to national surveys of newborns. Because the condition is X-linked recessive, most of those affected are hemizygous males. However, because of high gene frequency and parental consanguinity in some areas, female homozygosity accounts for nearly 10 percent of cases of G6PD deficiency. In addition, 10 percent of heterozygote females are G6PD deficient as a result of unequal X chromosome inactivation.

Oculocutaneous albinism

This is an autosomal recessive disorder affecting the pigmentation of skin, hair, and eyes. There are several types of oculocutaneous albinism: in the tyrosinase negative type, there is an absence of tyrosinase; in the tyrosinase positive type, the normal tyrosinase cannot enter pigment cells. The compound heterozygote is normal so the two forms are not allelic. This birth defect is rare in many parts of the world, but in subtropical Africa it ranks as the most prevalent single-gene disorder. The high risk of squamous cell carcinoma is the most serious consequence of oculocutaneous albinism. Early mortality from squamous cell carcinoma increases with proximity to the equator, resulting in the death of 90 percent of those affected in Nigeria and Tanzania before they reach age 30 (Luande et al., 1985). Additional symptoms of oculocutaneous albinism include photophobia, nystagmus, and squinting.

The prevalence of oculocutaneous albinism in subtropical Africa ranges from 1 in 1,000 (in an isolated cluster in the Tonga community of Zimbabwe) to between 1 per 3,900 and 1 per 5,000 in South Africa, Zimbabwe, and Nigeria (for selected prevalence studies in Africa, see Appendix A, Table A-6). These rates, which are two to four times those in European countries, may result from higher levels of parental consanguinity in certain African communities. Elevated rates of oculocutaneous albinism have also been noted in geographically isolated and consanguineous Latin American and Australian populations (Keeler, 1970; Okoro, 1975; Kromberg and Jenkins, 1982; Lund, 1996; Castilla and Sod, 1990).

Cystic fibrosis (CF)

A generalized disorder in which there is widespread dysfunction of the exocrine glands, characterized by signs of chronic pulmonary disease (due to excess mucus production in the respiratory tract), pancreatic deficiency, abnormally high levels of electrolytes in the sweat and occasionally by biliary cirrhosis. There is an ineffective immunologic defense against bacteria in the lungs. Without treatment, CF results in death for 95% of affected children before age 5. With diligent medical care patients with CF can survive beyond middle age. Although survival has improved in developed countries, CF often results in early mortality. The diagnosis of CF—complicated even in developed countries—requires tests for sweat chloride and, if positive, molecular screening to identify the mutation (Grody, 2001).

The frequency of CF varies considerably in different parts of the world and among different ethnic groups. A summary of prevalence rates of CF in several countries is presented in Appendix A (Table A-7). Reported birth prevalences range from a high of 1 per 2,000 births among Caucasians (Brock, 1996) to a low of 1 per 680,000 births (1 per 350,000 after 1980) among Japanese (Yamashiro et al., 1997). While sufficiently common among Caucasians to be one of the first diseases considered for genetic screening, CF has long been considered rare in non-Caucasian populations. Several lines of evidence argue against this conclusion, however. For example, CF was found to have a birth prevalence of 1 per 2,560 live births in Jordan (Nazer, 1992) and 1 per 3,000 live births in Turkey (Gurson et al., 1973). African-American CF patients were shown to have a different mutation profile from white CF patients; then a South African study identified different mutations in populations of African origin and predicted the incidence of CF to range from 1 in 784 to 1 in 13,924 births in this population (Padoa et al., 1999). In Africa, CF is thought to have been misdiagnosed as chronic pulmonary infection, tuberculosis, chronic diarrhea, and malnutrition. Thus, a lack of clinical awareness of the disorder and its misdiagnosis, rather than actual rarity, may explain the previous low CF prevalence reported in Africa (Padoa et al., 1999).

Phenylketonuria (PKU)

The congenital absence of phenylalanine hydroxylase (the enzyme that converts phenylalanine to tyrosine) is an autosomal recessive disorder. Phenylalanine accumulates in blood and seriously impairs early neuronal development. Affected neonates appear normal at birth but lose interest in their surroundings at 3 to 6 months of age and exhibit severe mental retardation by 1 year. Other clinical findings include an eczematous rash, microcephaly, growth retardation, and decreased pigmentation of hair and skin. A musty odor may be observed in the urine or sweat of individuals with PKU as a result of increased production of phenylpyruvate (Kietduriyakul et al., 1988; Cunningham, 2000).

Classical PKU affects 1 in 11,000 persons and is most prevalent among Caucasians (Eisensmith and Woo, 1994). In Turkey, the incidence of PKU is particularly high (1/4,370), largely as a result of consanguineous marriage (see Appendix A, Table A-8) (Ozalp et al., 1990).

Hemophilias A and B

The disease is characterized by subcutaneous and intramuscular hemorrhages, bleeding from the mouth, gums, lips and tongue, hematuria, and hemarthroses. Hemophilia A (classic hemophilia, factor VIII deficiency) is an X-linked disorder arising from deficiency of coagulation factor VIII, and hemophilia B (factor IX deficiency, Christmas disease), also X-linked, is due to deficiency of coagulation factor IX. Because of a sex-linked recessive inheritance pattern, if both parents are carriers for the disorder, male offspring will be affected by the disorder, and female offspring will be carriers (Kale, 1999). Extensive spontaneous bleeding is a lifelong burden, with physical, psychological, social, and financial repercussions (Kale, 1999). Hemophiliacs are at a high risk for HIV/AIDS and hepatitis B infection if blood products are contaminated (Handin, 1998). One in 5,000 males (1/10,000 for the total population) is born with deficiency or dysfunction of factor VIII (hemophilia A), and one in 50,000 males or in 100,000 total population is born with deficiency or dysfunction of factor IX (hemophilia B) (Handin, 1998).

BIRTH DEFECTS OF ENVIRONMENTAL ORIGIN

Exposure to a teratogen during embryonic or fetal life can cause functional disorders and malformations (Penchaszadeh, 1994; Polifka et al., 1996). The degree of teratogenicity of a given agent depends on its physical and chemical nature, as well as on the dose, route, and timing of exposure. Exposure to other agents and the biological susceptibility of the mother and embryo or fetus may also determine whether a particular exposure will produce damage (Polifka and Friedman, 1999). The major teratogens, listed in Table 2-2, include infectious pathogens, environmental toxins, recreational drugs, and medications.

TABLE 2-2 Teratogens and Their Effects on the Frequency of Malformations

Teratogen	Main Defects Caused	Estimated Risk
Infectious agents:		
Cytomegalovirus infection	Deafness; neurological damage; eye disorder	8% of maternal sero-conversion in pregnancy
Herpes simplex	Neurological damage; eye disorder; cutaneous scars	Not known
Rubella	Eye and heart defects; deafness; neurological damage	90% after serologically confirmed infection of mother in first 10 weeks of pregnancy
Toxoplasmosis	Neurological damage; eye disorder; deafness	30–40% after maternal seroconversion in pregnancy without treatment
Other maternal diseases:		
Phenylketonuria	Neurological damage; cardiac defects	Microcephaly in 8.5% of phenyketonuric infants with blood phenylalanine >1.2 nmol/L
Insulin-dependent diabetes mellitus	Cardiovascular and central nervous system (CNS) damage; caudal regression	Major defects in 8% of infants of affected women who did not receive special care during early pregnancy
Medications:		
Androgens and androgenic compounds	Anomalies of external genitalia	Clitoridal hypertrophy and virilization of female infants after first-trimester exposure at high doses; risks with other drugs not known but appear to be lower
Anticonvulsants	Spina bifida after valproate; oral clefts; cardiovascular defects	4% overall, but varies with number and nature of anticonvulsants used

(continued)

TABLE 2-2 continued

Teratogen	Main Defects Caused	Estimated Risk
Coumarin derivatives	Nasal hypoplasia; epiphyseal stippling; neurological damage	Nasal hypoplasia or epiphyseal stippling in 8% after use in first trimester; brain damage in 5% after use in second trimester
Diethylstilbestrol	Genital anomalies	Testicular anomalies, epididymal cysts, or penile hypoplasia in up to 20% of males, and ridges in cervix and/or vagina in up to 40% of females exposed to a dose of 150 mg between 7 and 34 weeks' gestation
Folic acid antagonists (aminopterin, methotrexate)	Craniofacial defects	40% after aminopterin in first 10 weeks of pregnancy; not known for methotrexate
Lithium	Cardiac defects, especially Ebstein's anomaly	3%
Retinoids	Microtia–anotia; CNS, cardioaortic, and thymic defects	20% after isotretinoin in first trimester
Thalidomide	Reduction deformities of limbs	50% after use in first 8 weeks of pregnancy
Recreational drugs: Cocaine	Urinary tract defects	Major defects in 5% of users of cocaine with or without other drugs
Alcohol	Neurological damage; cardiac and joint defects	30% of infants of women with manifest chronic alcoholism
Environmental pollutants: Methylmercury	Neurological damage	6% of infants in fishing village where seafood was contaminated
Miscellaneous: Iodine deficiency	Neurological damage; deafness	40% of surviving infants in iodine-deficient area whose mothers' blood total thyroxine was <25 ng/mL
Ionizing radiation	Neurological damage	Microcephaly in 70% after estimated dose >1.5 gy from atomic bombs in first 18 weeks of pregnancy

SOURCE: Adapted from Leck, 1994.

Infectious Pathogens

Infections during pregnancy are common, and the majority of maternal infections do not affect the fetus. Those that do, however, can result in fetal loss or severe birth defects. Teratogenic pathogens may exert their effects immediately, or they may initiate complex processes that cause damage throughout gestation and into infancy (Alford and Pass, 1981; Hanshaw, 1985). Although infections cause only a fraction of total birth defects, they represent an opportunity for reducing birth defects through prevention (Hanshaw, 1985).

A variety of agents can infect the fetus or newborn either in utero or intrapartum and cause birth defects and/or injury to developing organs—particularly the brain, eye, and ear—with lifelong sequelae among survivors. The most important agents are rubella virus, cytomegalovirus, *Toxoplasma gondii,* and herpes simplex virus. Infectious pathogens, such as syphilis, can cause congenital infections that result in postpartum conditions (e.g., bone deformities, developmental disorders, blindness, deafness (Finelli et al., 1998) if left untreated. These are addressed in a companion report (Institute of Medicine, 2003). Specific diagnoses may be difficult because some agents (e.g., cytomegalovirus, *Toxoplasma gondii*) produce similar clinical syndromes and because infection may be asymptomatic or not clinically obvious at birth. Laboratory diagnosis or confirmation of a clinically suspected infection may be difficult or impossible in some developing-country settings.

Infectious pathogens are distributed worldwide; prevalence data from developing countries are limited, however, because of the difficulties in diagnosis. Nonetheless, it is known that for many agents, the risk of maternal infection during pregnancy—and therefore of fetal or neonatal infection—varies with socioeconomic status, access to preventive and curative health services (especially immunization), prevalence of sexually transmitted diseases (STDs), cultural practices, and geographic region. The following discussion of these disorders draws on the limited number of studies on infection-associated birth defects in developing countries and on developed country data for the symptoms and understanding of risk factors.

Rubella

Maternal infection with rubella virus in early gestation interferes with critical organ development in the fetus. The resulting birth defects—blindness, deafness, cardiovascular anomalies, and mental retardation—are referred to collectively as congenital rubella syndrome (CRS). The prognosis for infants with severe CRS is poor. For those diagnosed during the first year, mortality is high, and most survivors are seriously impaired (Bos et al., 1995).

Since 1969, vaccination against rubella has made CRS increasingly rare in most developed countries. Rubella remains endemic in many developing countries, however, as shown in Figure 2-3. Although it is a major cause of preventable hearing impairment and blindness, CRS is often not recognized or recorded (Tantivanich et al., 1980; Cutts and Vynnycky, 1999; Lawn et al., 2000; St. John and Benjamin, 2000). The majority of all women of childbearing age have acquired immunity to rubella virus by exposure or vaccination (Banatvala, 1998), but there appears to be considerable variability in maternal immunity, as well as in CRS incidence, among countries (see Table 2-3).

A model of rubella incidence predicts about 236,000 cases of CRS annually in nonepidemic years, mostly in developing countries; the number of cases may increase tenfold during epidemics (Salisbury and Savinykh, 1991; Banatvala, 1998). In unimmunized populations, rubella epidemics occur on average every 4 to 7 years (Cutts et al., 1997). Over the last 25 years, surveillance of these epidemics has documented CRS birth prevalence rates of 0.6–2.2 (Banatvala, 1998) and 0.6–4.1 (World Health Organization, 2000) per 1,000 live births. These rates are similar to those reported

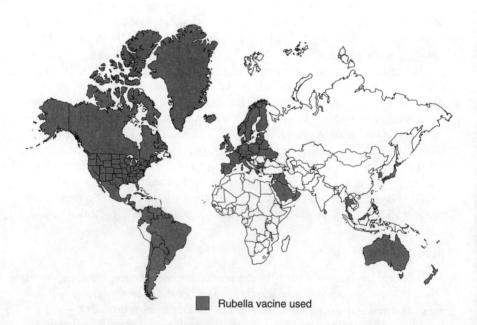

Rubella vacine used

FIGURE 2-3 Countries/areas with rubella vaccine in their national immunization program, April 2000.
SOURCE: World Health Organization, 2000.

TABLE 2-3 Frequency of Congenital Rubella Syndrome and Rubella Susceptibility in Pregnant Women

Country (city)	CRS Birth Prevalence	Proportion of Adult Women Susceptible
India, Lucknow	Case-control study showed rubella IgG[a] in 62% of 55 children with CRS-compatible malformations vs. 10% of control children (Chaturvedi et al., 1976).	15–22% (Mathur et al., 1974, 1982)
India, New Delhi	Rubella confirmed in 7–12% of infants with suspect congenital infection (Manjunath and Balaya, 1984; Broor et al., 1991).	>30% (Khare et al., 1987; Satpathy, 1989; Khare et al., 1990)
Israel	CRS birth prevalence 1.7 per 1,000 live births in 1972. Among women pregnant in 1972, 4.7% had clinical rubella, and 6.4% had subclinical infection (Fogel et al., 1976).	25% (Fogel et al., 1976)
Jamaica	Average CRS birth prevalence 0.4 per 1,000 live births over 10 years (Baxter, 1986).	43% (urban), 51% (rural) (Dowdle et al., 1970), 42% (Lam, 1972)
Malaysia	35% of 165 deaf children had rubella pigmentary retinopathy (Elango et al., 1994). In infants, 221 cases of CRS were identified through screening for *toxoplasmosis*, other infections, *rubella, cytomegalovirus* infection, and *herpes simplex* (Tan, 1985).	42% (Lam, 1972)
Oman	CRS birth prevalence 0.5 per 1,000 live births in 1988 (33); 0.7 per 1,000 in 1993 (Expanded Programme on Immunization, 1994).	8% in 1988–1989 (4 to 30% in different regions) (Expanded Programme on Immunization, 1994)
Nigeria, Ibadan	9 of 41 cases of patent ductus arteriosus, CRS-associated (Antia, 1974).	30% (Odelola, 1978)
Panama	CRS birth prevalence 2.2 per 1,000 live births in 1986 outbreak and 30% of rubella cases in women of childbearing age (Owens and Espino, 1989).	38% (urban), 64% (rural) (Dowdle et al., 1970)
Singapore	CRS birth prevalence 1.5 per 1,000 live births in 1969 outbreak (Tan et al., 1970).	47% (Doraisingham and Goh, 1981)
Sri Lanka	CRS birth prevalence 0.9 per 1,000 live births in 1994–1995 outbreak (Gunasekera and Gunasekera, 1996).	43% (Mendis, 1989)
Thailand	56% of 49 infants with suspect intrauterine infections were rubella-IgM-positive (Tantivanich et al., 1980).	32–36% (Phiromsawat et al., 1988; Pruksananonda and Bumrungtrakul, 1983)
Trinidad and Tobago	CRS birth prevalence 0.6 per 1,000 live births in 1982–1983 outbreak (Ali et al., 1986).	68% (Dowdle et al., 1970)

[a]Ig = immunoglobulin.

SOURCE: Cutts et al., 1997.

for developed countries during the prevaccination era. Even higher rates are found in CRS prevalence studies with follow-up after 2 or more years, since this is the time when signs such as deafness or psychomotor retardation are more likely to be detected.

Cytomegalovirus (CMV)

CMV is the most common intrauterine infection and is estimated to affect 0.4–2.5 percent of live-born infants. Over 90 percent of the infected infants are asymptomatic at birth, but 5–17 percent of them will later develop sensorineural hearing loss, chorioretinitis, mental retardation, and neurological damage. Nearly 90 percent of the infants with symptoms at birth will develop severe abnormalities associated with damage to the central nervous system (CNS) or sensory organs. (Alford et al, 1990; Fowler et al., 1992; Stagno and Whitley, 1985).

Like other members of the herpes family, CMV can persist in a latent state following a primary infection. Despite maternal immunity, it can be reactivated during pregnancy and transmitted to the fetus, or reinfection can occur from a different strain of CMV (Bos et al., 1995). The infection is, however, generally less severe in the presence of maternal antibody (Stagno et al., 1984).

The average age of CMV infection in a population depends on the level of hygiene, which in turn is related to the level of development. In countries with high standards of hygiene, fewer women of childbearing age are immune to CMV, putting the fetus at greater risk. In studies from developing countries, almost all women of childbearing age have been found to be immune: 96 percent in South Korea (Sohn et al., 1992), 100 percent in Thailand (Taechowisan et al., 1997), 99 percent in Turkey (Hizel et al., 1999), 88 percent in the Gambia (Bello and Whittle, 1991), 100 percent in the Ivory Coast (Stagno et al., 1982), and 60–100 percent in South Africa (Stagno et al., 1984). The percentages of neonates with CMV vary: 0.2–2.3 percent in South Africa (Stagno et al., 1984), 1.4 percent in the Ivory Coast (Stagno et al., 1982), and 1 percent in South Korea (Sohn et al., 1992).

Toxoplasma gondii

This infection is generally transmitted by oocysts present in soil or water that has been contaminated by the feces of infected cats or by tissue cysts that persist in the undercooked meat of infected animals (Cook et al., 2000; Dubey, 2000). The seroprevalence of toxoplasmosis in women during pregnancy has been found to vary markedly in different populations: 12 percent in Thailand (Chintana et al., 1991), 14 percent in Indonesia (Gandahusada, 1991), 25 percent in Egypt (Essawy et al., 1990), 35 percent in

Tanzania (Doehring et al., 1995), and 75–80 percent in Nigeria (Onadeko, 1996).

The signs and symptoms of congenital toxoplasmosis include chorioretinitis, anemia, jaundice, hepatomegaly, splenomegaly, intracranial calcifications, hydrocephalus or microcephaly, and growth restriction. Long-term sequelae include mental retardation, seizures, severe visual impairment, blindness, and hearing impairment.

Herpes simplex virus (HSV)

Genital herpes is becoming a leading cause of genital ulcers in many developing countries (O'Farrell, 1999). Herpes simplex virus types 1 (HSV-1) and 2 (HSV-2) can cause genital infection and be transmitted from mother to fetus or newborn. HSV infection in the newborn can be acquired in utero (rare), intrapartum (most common), and postnatally. The newborn is at greatest risk if the mother has a primary HSV infection at or near the time of delivery (transmission rates of 50 percent or more) (Brown et al., 1997). Unfortunately, many women are asymptomatic at the time of primary infection. Neonatal HSV infection is a life-threatening illness that presents clinically as isolated CNS disease; disseminated disease with CNS involvement; or isolated skin, eye, and/or mouth infection. CNS damage, including microcephaly, hydranencephaly, and/or meningoencephalitis, can result. Therapy with intravenous acyclovir reduces the risk of death (0 percent for localized skin disease, 5 percent for encephalitis, 25 percent for disseminated disease), but morbidity remains high. While 95 percent of those with skin disease are normal at 2 years of age, only 40 percent of those surviving encephalitis and 60 percent of those surviving disseminated disease are normal at age two (Whitley at al., 1991).

Genital herpes is increasingly being recognized as an important problem in developing countries (Carey and Handsfield, 2000). Few studies of HSV during pregnancy have been conducted in developing countries, but maternal seroprevalences of 50 percent for HSV-1 and 20 percent for HSV-2 have been reported in India (Kaur et al., 1999); in Eritrea, 97 percent of pregnant women were found to be seropositive for HSV-1 and 23 percent for HSV-2 (Ghebrekidan et al., 1999); in Costa Rica, 97 percent were seropositive for HSV-1 and 39 percent for HSV-2 (Oberle et al., 1989). In a large study of the seroepidemiology of HSV infections in many countries, Nahmias et al. (1990) reported that adult populations in several countries, including Rwanda, Zaire, Senegal, China, Taiwan, Haiti, Jamaica, and Costa Rica, had a prevalence of HSV-1 antibodies of 85 percent. Rates of HSV-2 antibodies among pregnant women varied from less than 10 percent in Japan, Italy, and Spain to 50 percent in Haiti. Nahmias et al. noted an increase in HSV-2 seroprevalence rates over time.

Other Maternal Illnesses

Insulin-dependent diabetes mellitus (IDDM)

This affects about 0.5 percent of pregnancies in developed countries and is reported to be equally prevalent in several developing countries. Pregnant women with preexisting diabetes are at risk for having infants with CNS, cardiovascular, renal, and limb defects (Khoury et al., 1989; Loffredo et al., 2001). Such pregnancies also have higher-than-average rates of fetal loss and stillbirth.

Phenylketonuria

This is an autosomal recessive disorder carrying a significant risk that affected infants will also have disorder, a congenital malformation, or neurological impairment (see the earlier discussion under single-gene disorders). Improved outcomes have been reported for infants when their mothers maintain low-phenylalanine diets (Cunningham, 2000; Platt et al., 2000).

Hyperthermia

This involves a fever of 39°C or higher for at least 24 hours during the first 4 weeks of pregnancy. It increases the risk for NTDs and other birth defects (Kalter and Warkany, 1983; Warkany, 1986; Chambers et al., 1998; Graham et al., 1998). It is not known whether these birth defects are due to the hyperthermia or the underlying cause of the fever.

Maternal Nutrition

Deficiencies in maternal nutrition, particularly of folate and iodine, during pregnancy can increase the risk of an infant's being born with a birth defect.

Folic acid deficiency

When this occurs before and during the early weeks of pregnancy, it has been shown by randomized controlled trials to be the predominant cause of NTDs (spina bifida, anencephaly, and encephalocele) (MRC Vitamin Study Research Group, 1991; Czeizel and Dudas, 1992). The number of children born each year with spina bifida and anencephaly is estimated at 300,000 or more. Further discussion follows in the section in this chapter on NTDs.

Iodine deficiency disorders (IDDs)

These occur worldwide and are among the most readily preven causes of birth defects (Hollowell and Hannon, 1997; Maberly, 1998, in 1990, it was estimated that 43 million people worldwide live with cretinism, mental retardation, and brain damage due to IDD (United Nations Children's Fund, 1998). In endemic areas, where up to 100 percent of the population fails to consume adequate iodine (Ali, 1995; Wyss et al., 1996; Yusuf et al., 1996; Geelhoed, 1999; Kouame et al., 1998), nearly every developing fetus is affected by IDD (Mittal et al., 2000). Severe maternal iodine deficiency begins to affect the fetus in the second trimester of pregnancy, and the resulting damage becomes irreversible at the end of that period (DeLong et al., 1985). The spectrum of these disorders includes endemic cretinism, endemic goiter, and reduced intellectual ability.

Cretins have severe mental retardation, with IQ usually below 30 (Boyages et al., 1987; Sankar et al., 1998). They have broad CNS defects that include preservation of primitive reflexes, deafness, squint, a characteristic grin, and spasticity that affects the larger proximal limb muscles more than the distal extremities (DeLong et al., 1985). They also have cartilage defects, bony deformities, and laxity in joints. If they are able to walk, it is with difficulty. The presence or absence of goiter, stunted growth and sexual development, and gross myxedema depends on the severity of the condition and the time lived with congenital hypothyroidism. Lifelong hypothyroidism in certain individuals substantially alters the clinical picture (Halpern et al., 1991). Endemic cretinism occurs in areas severely deficient in iodine and has been reported to affect 0.5–11 percent of the population in several countries (Wyss et al., 1996; Yusuf et al., 1996; Jalil et al., 1997; Bellis et al., 1998; Kouame et al., 1998; Sankar et al., 1998; Geelhoed, 1999). A rural hospital study in Zaire that examined more than 3400 consecutive births found 5 percent of the neonates to be cretins (Smith et al., 1986).

Endemic goiter is the hallmark of iodine deficiency and has been used as an indicator of deficiency in a population when goiter rates in school-age children exceed 5 percent. Even after the introduction of iodized salt to a deficient population, goiters may persist for many years despite adequate iodine intake (World Health Organization, 2001). Goiter rates can approach 100 percent in severely iodine-deficient populations, but a rate of 40–60 percent is more common. The presence or absence of goiter in an individual does not relate directly to the level of iodine deficiency, associated perturbations of thyroid function, or other features of IDD (Maberly and Eastman, 1976).

In populations with mild to moderately severe iodine deficiency, population cognitive performance distribution curves are shifted by as much as one standard deviation as compared with iodine-replete populations (Stanbury, 1994). A meta-analysis of 18 studies involving 2,214 individuals examined cognitive and neuromotor function (Bleichrodt et al., 1980). The mean IQ scores in the iodine-deficient group were 13.5 points lower than in the control group. This would suggest that the widespread effect of iodine deficiency on brain function and learning ability has profound implications for the economic and manpower development of affected populations (Dunn, 1994).

Medications

A number of therapeutic drugs have been implicated as teratogens. Teratogenicity is dependent on the timing of use in pregnancy, dose levels, genetic susceptibility, and other factors. The use of medications during pregnancy is of particular concern in the developing world because of the widespread over-the-counter availability of many drugs, as well as the large proportion of unplanned pregnancies and the fact that most women are unaware of their pregnancies during the first few weeks. Teratogenic medications that are important in developing countries are reviewed below; additional drugs with proven teratogenic effects in humans are listed in Table 2-4. New drugs are rarely tested in pregnant women, so their description includes a disclaimer such as "use in pregnancy is not recommended unless the potential benefits justify the potential risks to the fetus." Common drugs initially thought to be teratogenic but subsequently proven safe include diazepam, oral contraceptives, spermicides, salicylates, and Bendectin (doxylamine plus pyridoxine) (Koren et al., 1998). Alternative drugs that are not known to be teratogenic are listed in Table 2-5.

Thalidomide

This is the paradigm of teratogenic drugs. It was withdrawn from global markets in the early 1960s when it was determined that the sedative—then commonly prescribed for morning sickness—had caused severe limb and organ defects in more than 8,000 infants in 46 countries (Koren et al., 1998; Vanchieri, 1997; Grover et al., 2000). Today, because of its additional properties as an immunomodulator, thalidomide is once again available in many countries for indications including leprosy and HIV (Castilla et al., 1996; Diggle, 2001). Access to thalidomide is likely to result in birth defects unless preventive measures are established to protect pregnant women from exposure (Vanchieri, 1997; Annas and Elias, 1999). For example, 34 infants have been born with thalidomide embryopathy in the last 25 years in areas of South America where leprosy is endemic (Castilla et al., 1996).

TABLE 2-4 Drugs with Proven Teratogenic Effects in Humans[a]

Drug	Teratogenic Effect
Aminopterin,[b] methotrexate	Central nervous system (CNS) and limb malformation
Angiotensin-converting enzyme inhibitors	Prolonged renal failure in neonates, decreased skull ossification, renal tubular dysgenesis
Anticholinergic drugs	Neonatal meconium ileus
Antithyroid drugs (propylthiouracil and methimazole)	Fetal and neonatal goiter and hypothyroidism, aplasia cutis (with methimazole)
Carbamazepine	Neural tube defects (NTDs)
Cyclophosphamide	CNS malformations, secondary cancer
Danazol and other androgenic drugs	Masculinization of female fetuses
Diethylstilbestrol[b]	Vaginal carcinoma and other genitourinary defects in female and male offspring
Hypoglycemic drugs	Neonatal hypoglycemia
Lithium	Ebstein's anomaly
Misoprostol	Moebius sequence
Nonsteroidal anti-inflammatory drugs	Constriction of the ductus arteriosus,[c] necrotizing enterocolitis
Paramethadione[b]	Facial and CNS defects
Phenytoin	Growth retardation, CNS defects
Psychoactive drugs (e.g., barbiturates, opioids, benzodiazepines)	Neonatal withdrawal syndrome when drug is taken in late pregnancy
Systemic retinoids (isoretinoin and etretinate)	CNS, craniofacial, cardiovascular, and other defects
Tetracycline	Anomalies of teeth and bone
Thalidomide	Limb-shortening defects, internal organ defects
Trimethadione[b]	Facial and CNS defects
Valproic acid	NTDs
Warfarin	Skeletal and CNS defects, Dandy-Walker syndrome

[a]Only drugs that are teratogenic when used at clinically recommended doses are listed. The list includes all drugs proven to affect neonatal morphology or brain development and some of the toxic manifestations predicted on the basis of the pharmacologic actions of the drugs.
[b]The drug is not currently in clinical use.
[c]Sulindac probably does not have this effect.
SOURCE: Briggs et al., 1994.

Misoprostol

This is used for cervical ripening and induction of labor, also to induce early abortion (Gonzalez et al., 1998; Orioli and Castilla, 2000). The drug is not always effective for this purpose, and surviving newborns have exhibited several birth defects attributed to vascular disruption, including transverse limb reduction anomalies, constriction rings, Moebius sequence, hy-

TABLE 2-5 Drugs of Choice for Pregnant Women: Selected Drugs Not Known to Be Teratogenic

Condition	Drugs of Choice	Alternative Drugs	Comments
Acne	*Topical:* erythromycin, clindamycin, benzoyl peroxide	*Systemic:* erythromycin *Topical:* tretinoin (vitamin A acid)	Isotretinoin is contraindicated.
Allergic rhinitis	*Topical:* glucocorticoids, cromolyn, decongestants, xylometazoline, oxymetazoline, naphazoline, phenylephrine *Systemic:* diphenhydramine, dimenhydrinate, tripelennamin, astemizole		
Constipation	Docusate sodium, calcium, glycerine, sorbitol, lactulose, mineral oil, magnesium hydroxide	Bisacodyl, phenolphthalein	
Cough	Diphenhydramine, codeine, dextromethorphan		
Depression	Tricyclic antidepressant drugs, fluoxetine	Lithium	When lithium is used in first trimester, fetal echocardiography and ultrasonograpy are recommended because of small risk of cardiovascular defects.
Diabetes	Insulin (human)	Insulin (beef or pork)	Hypoglycemic drugs should be avoided.
Headache, tension	Acetaminophen	Aspirin and nonsteroidal anti-inflammatory drugs, benzodiazepines	Aspirin and nonsteroidal anti-inflammatory drugs should be avoided in third trimester.
Migraine	Acetaminophen, codeine, dimenhydrinate	α-Adrenergic-receptor antagonists and tricyclic antidepressant drugs (for prophylaxis)	Limited experience with ergotamine has not revealed evidence of teratogenicity, but there is concern about potent

Condition			
Hypertension	Labetalol, methyldopa	β-Adrenergic-receptor antagonists, prazosin, hydralazine	vasoconstriction and uterine contraction. Angiotensin-converting enzyme inhibitors should be avoided because of risk of severe neonatal renal insufficiency.
Hyperthyroidism	Propylthiouracil	β-Adrenergic-receptor antagonists (for symptoms)	
Mania (and bipolar affective disorder)	Lithium, chlorpromazine, haloperidol	For depressive episodes: tricyclic antidepressants drugs, fluoxetine, valproic acid	If lithium is used in first trimester, fetal echocardiography and ultrasonography are recommended because of small risk of cardiac anomalies; valproic acid may be given after neural tube closure is complete.
Nausea, vomiting, motion sickness	Diclectin (doxylamine plus pyridoxine)	Chlorpromazine, metoclopramide (in third trimester), diphenhydramine, dimenhydrinate, meclizine, cyclizine	
Peptic ulcer disease	Antacids, magnesium hydroxide, aluminum hydroxide, calcium carbonate, ranitidine	Sucralfate, bismuth subsalicylate *Topical:* local anesthetics	
Pruritus	*Topical:* moisturizing creams or lotions, aluminum acetate, zinc oxide cream or ointment, calamine lotion, glucocorticoids *Systemic:* hydroxyzine, diphenhydramine, glucocorticoides, astemizole		
Thrombophlebitis, deep-vein thrombosis	Heparin, antifibrinolytic drugs, streptokinase		Streptokinase is associated with a risk of bleeding; warfarin should be avoided.

SOURCE: Smith et al., 1994.

drocephalus, and arthrogryposis (Gonzalez et al., 1998; Orioli and Castilla, 2000). A multicenter, case-controlled study conducted in Brazil showed that 34 percent of mothers of infants with vascular disruption defects had taken misoprostol during the prenatal period, compared with only 4 percent in a control group consisting of mothers of children with other birth defects (Vargas et al., 2000). Another Brazilian study of 15 patients with growth retardation, underdeveloped bones, joint rigidity, and short feet with equinovarus revealed that all their mothers had taken 400–4800 micrograms of misoprostol between the eighth and twelfth weeks of pregnancy (Coelho et al., 2000).

Anticonvulsant drugs

When used during pregnancy, these have been associated with congenital anomalies. Phenobarbital, phenytoin, carbamazepine, and valproate have been implicated as causes of major malformations, including NTDs, microcephaly, growth restriction, and minor malformations of the face and fingers (Koren, 1998; Samren, 1999; Arpino et al., 2000; Adab et al., 2001; Holmes et al., 2001). These birth defects do not appear to be associated with maternal epilepsy itself (Holmes et al., 2001). A large retrospective cohort study has concluded that antiepileptic drugs used in polytherapy carry a higher risk of causing birth defects than those used in monotherapy (Samren et al., 1999). Research is under way to explore the effectiveness and risk of monotherapy for epilepsy in pregnant women (Adab et al., 2001).

Anticoagulants

When used during pregnancy, anticoagulants cause congenital disorders. Fetal exposure, particularly during the first trimester, to derivatives of coumarin such as Coumadin (warfarin) can cause nasal hypoplasia, stippling of bones, optic atrophy, microcephaly, and growth and mental retardation. Exposure after the first trimester has also been associated with facial anomalies and fetal and neonatal hemorrhage. Heparin is the preferred anticoagulant for use during pregnancy because it does not cross the placenta (Hardman et al., 1996).

Alcohol and Recreational Drugs

Alcohol

Heavy alcohol use during pregnancy is associated with fetal alcohol syndrome (FAS) and alcohol-related neurodevelopmental disorder (ARND) in exposed children. FAS/ARND has been reported in up to 9 per 1,000 infants exposed to high alcohol levels during pregnancy (Sampson et al., 1997). FAS encompasses a constellation of physical abnormalities, including alterations in facial features and fetal growth reduction, as well as behavioral and cognitive effects (Institute of Medicine, 1996). With or without the recognized dysmorphologic pattern known as FAS, mental retardation is the most serious and constant effect of alcohol use during pregnancy. Research to measure the prevalence of FAS in South African school children is described in Box 2-3.

BOX 2-3 Fetal Alcohol Syndrome (FAS) in South Africa

The occurrence of FAS in the traditional wine-growing area of Western Cape Province, South Africa, was first documented in 1978. An initial study of 636 women who voluntarily attended 17 antenatal clinics in three regions determined that 43 percent of the pregnant women reported varying degrees of alcohol consumption during their current pregnancy. Nearly one-quarter of the women reported an alcohol intake sufficient to place their unborn child at high risk for FAS. Alcohol consumption during pregnancy was more frequent for rural than urban women. Women who drank heavily tended to follow a pattern of binge drinking over weekends, and 30 percent of those interviewed also smoked tobacco (Croxford and Viljoen, 1999; Viljoen, 1999).

An epidemiological study to determine the prevalence of FAS in a Western Cape community of schoolchildren used active case ascertainment (Institute of Medicine, 1996) to study 992 children in their first year at 12 of 13 local schools. Most of the children were of African or mixed (Khoisan, African, Malay, and Caucasian) ancestry. The age-specific (6–7 years) prevalence of FAS in this community was about 48 per 1,000, the highest yet reported. The study did not provide the birth prevalence of FAS, since the infant mortality rate in the Western Cape is 30 per 1,000 live births. The data also showed that 61 percent of the FAS children were from rural areas (May et al., 2000). The significant risk factors for FAS in this low socioeconomic group were maternal educational attainment, low religiosity, current family drinking history, current use of alcohol, drinking before pregnancy, total alcohol consumption, smoking, gravidity, and parity (Viljoen et al., 2001).

This study was the first in the developing world to use active case ascertainment to estimate the prevalence of FAS. This syndrome had not previously been recognized as a problem in South Africa (Christianson et al., 2000). More recently, the same methodology has been applied to study 834 school entry children in four South African communities in Gauteng Province. The communities were selected to represent a spectrum of ethnic groups living in poverty, among whom alcohol abuse was reportedly common (Viljoen and Craig, 2001). The combined age-specific prevalence of FAS in these communities was 18 per 1,000.

Tobacco

Evidence for the role of smoking in birth defects is controversial. The well-established role of smoking in preterm births and intrauterine growth restriction is discussed in the companion to this report (Institute of Medicine, 2003).

Environmental Pollutants

Although teratogenic pollutants are known to be present in some developing-country settings and have been associated with birth defects in clinical studies, their impact in developing countries remains unknown. Common teratogens may include heavy metals such as organic mercury, pesticides such as DDT, solvents, and other toxic contaminants (Jacobson and Jacobson, 1996; Ramsay and Reynolds, 2000). This risk is poorly defined because most developing countries do not have systems to detect exposures or resulting problems, nor do they have laws to protect against hazardous exposure. Research is needed to establish whether these pollutants contribute significantly to the occurrence of birth defects in different settings.

Mercury contamination of the environment can be widespread and persistent (Institute of Medicine, 2000). Methylmercury causes birth defects in the central nervous system and, to a lesser extent, in the liver and kidneys (Institute of Medicine, 2000). The chemical accumulates up the food chain and may be present at teratogenic levels in some fish populations. Mass methylmercury poisoning, which occurred in Japan in the 1950s (Friberg et al., 1971) and in Iraq in the 1970s (Marsh et al., 1987), resulted in severe neurological dysfunction and developmental abnormalities among children who were exposed in utero. The adverse effects included mental retardation, cerebral palsy, deafness, blindness, and dysarthria.

Occupational exposure to environmental pollutants, both agricultural and industrial, can be teratogenic or fetotoxic. The risk posed by maternal occupational exposures to industrial pollutants is unknown, and male-mediated teratogenesis remains controversial (McDonald et al., 1989; Olshan et al., 1990).

Ionizing Radiation

Studies of atomic bomb survivors demonstrated that exposure to ionizing radiation during gestation can damage the developing brain, particularly when exposure occurs 8 to 25 weeks after ovulation (Schull and Otake, 1999). Diagnostic radiography involves a low level of X-ray expo-

sure of the fetus so that, with protection, the risk of a bir
(Fattibene et al., 1999; Fenig et al., 2001).

52

BIRTH DEFECTS OF COMPLEX AND UNKNOWN

The origins of most birth defects have not been establish   ..y of
them are thought to be due to the additive effects of a few (oligogenic) or
many (polygenic) genes, which may interact with nongenetic (environmental) factors. These conditions are usually limited to a single organ system
and include the following: NTDs, congenital heart disease, cleft lip and
palate, talipes or clubfoot, and developmental dysplasia of the hip. These
conditions were selected for discussion because of their documented disease
burden in developing countries.

Neural Tube Defects

These encompass a range of congenital malformations that result from
incomplete development of the brain and spinal cord or their protective
coverings. The three major types are anencephaly, spina bifida, and
encephalocele.

Spina bifida is the incomplete closure of the neural tube, which is the
predecessor of the spinal cord. The birth outcome varies with the location
of the genetic defect and whether it affects the neural tube, skeletal components, and/or skin. In some cases, the affected infant is born with the spinal
cord exposed on the surface as a neural plaque, and it may include
meningeal tissue. This interrupted development of the spinal cord occurs in
the first 4 to 5 weeks of fetal development and causes serious clinical
problems that may include hydrocephalus, paralysis, incontinence, or skeletal deformities depending on the location and nature of the defect. Although spina bifida has long been considered to be a lethal condition,
surgery at birth saves some infants, but they may be significantly handicapped (Shibuya and Murray, 1998; Gross et al., 1983; Hunt, 1990;
Laurence 1974; McLaughlin et al., 1985). In resource-poor situations, the
future of an affected child is severely compromised.

Anencephaly is the congenital absence of the cranial vault with cerebral
hemispheres missing or reduced to small masses attached to the base of the
skull. This condition causes significant mortality before and soon after
birth.

Encephalocele involves a protrusion of the brain and its covering membranes through the skull. This condition may or may not be lethal, but
serious neurological deficits usually occur.

Worldwide, NTDs are estimated to affect 300,000 or more infants each year (Murray and Lopez, 1998). The wide variation in birth prevalence of NTDs, demonstrated in Appendix A (Table A-9), can be explained by genetic and nutritional factors and in part by differences in the availability of prenatal screening and termination of affected pregnancies (Shibuya and Murray, 1998). Epidemiological studies show a strong association between NTDs and inadequate maternal consumption of folic acid during the periconceptional period (see the discussion of folic acid deficiency in Chapter 3). Mutations of the methylenetetrahydrofolate reductase gene in the absence of a folate-rich diet are associated with elevated maternal plasma homocysteine and increased risk of NTDs in offspring (Wilcken, 1997; Van der Put et al, 1998).

Congenital Heart Disease

A malformation of the heart or large blood vessels near the heart is present at birth. This is the most common of the major birth defects, affecting 8 per 1,000 live births, and is a leading cause of birth defect-related deaths, despite improvements in diagnosis and surgical treatments over the last 40 years. The more serious symptoms and signs of congenital heart disease include cyanosis, pulmonary hypertension, growth retardation, and syncope. Left untreated, these symptoms will, in most cases, prove fatal before age 20 (Cartmill et al., 1966; Rygg et al., 1971; Kirklin and Barrat-Boyes, 1993; Cohen et al., 2001). Today, echocardiography, available in urban centers in developing countries, can provide a reliable anatomical diagnosis when clinical data suggest a cardiac defect.

A variety of conditions—maternal rubella infection, maternal diabetes, alcohol abuse, genetic abnormalities, and chromosomal disorders such as Down syndrome—can result in congenital cardiac malformations. Lesions include ventricular septal defect, atrial septal defect, pulmonary stenosis, coarctation of the aorta, aortic stenosis, and tetralogy of Fallot. Prevalence data on congenital heart disease (both the general disease and specific lesions) in developing countries are given in Appendix A (Table A-10). Because congenital heart disease is often not recognizable at birth, studies have used a wide range of ascertainment methods (Shibuya and Murray, 1998).

Cleft Lip and/or Cleft Palate

These are congenital malformations involving a gap in the soft palate and roof of the mouth, sometimes extending through the upper lip. This condition occurs when the various parts of a lip or palate don't grow together to make a single lip or hard palate. It is usually correctable. Affected infants have difficulty first with feeding, then with speech development, hearing, and tooth formation; stigmatization and discrimination pose lifelong problems. Malnutrition and infection resulting from cleft lip and/or palate can lead to severe illness and, in some cases, death (Shibuya and Murray, 1998). Half of all infants with cleft lip and/or palate have additional birth defects, such as heart malformations, that co-occur as genetic syndromes (Shibuya and Murray, 1998).

Birth prevalence rates for oral clefts from several countries are shown in Appendix A (Table A-11); most lie between 1 and 2 per 1,000 live births. Several of the studies listed in the appendix identified environmental, maternal, and birth-order risk factors for these congenital malformations (Choudhury et al., 1989; Wu et al., 1995; Chuangsuwanich et al., 1998; Cooper et al., 2000).

Talipes or Clubfoot

This involves a spectrum of common abnormalities in ankle joints and in the bones, muscles, and ligaments of the foot. The main types of deformities include abduction of the whole foot with plantar inversion, external rotation of the foot, concave profile of the sole, convex profile of the sole, and medial deviation of the anterior third of the foot (Winter et al., 1988). Pathological changes resulting from the deformity vary among patients. In severe cases, bones may be smaller than normal, with displacement of the talocalcaneonavicular joint. When bones are normal in shape and size, the deformity is maintained by contracted muscles, tendons, and ligaments (Sinha, 1987). Transient deformities not requiring treatment are not considered here.

Left untreated, talipes prevents normal motion of the foot and produces an awkward gait. If both feet are affected (about 50 percent of cases), the child is forced to walk on the balls of the feet or, when the feet are badly twisted, on the sides or even the tops of the feet. These surfaces often become infected and develop large, hard calluses. Over time, talipes causes arthritis and can hinder the growth of the entire leg.

The birth prevalence of talipes in several populations is presented in Appendix A (Table A-12). The rate in most countries is 1.5 to 4 per 1,000 live births. Some 30–40 percent of infants with talipes have other severe congenital malformations, particularly spina bifida. The etiology of talipes is heterogeneous and complex, and involves the interplay of extrinsic intrauterine compression (Dietz, 1985); intrinsic neurological deficit (Nadeem et al., 2000); and genetic anomalies, including major genes (Yang et al., 1987).

Developmental Dysplasia of the Hip (DDH)

A malformation of the hip joint in which the head of the femur is not correctly positioned in the acetabulum. The cause is unknown, but genetic factors may play a role. Problems range from the relatively rare congenital dislocation of the hip where the head of the femur is completely outside the acetabulum and the hip is very unstable to conditions where the displacement shortens one leg and causes limping, joint and knee problems, pain, and the degenerative changes of osteoarthrosis (Leck, 2000).

The prevalence reported for DDH varies widely (see Appendix A, Table A-13), due more to the criteria applied, rather than to actual differences among populations (Dunn et al., 1985; Herring, 1990; Bialik et al., 1999). However, two recent hospital-based studies conducted by experienced diagnosticians using both manual and ultrasound methods—one in Singapore (Ang et al., 1997), the other in Israel (Bialik et al., 1999)—reported birth prevalence rates for DDH of about 5 per 1,000 live births. Females outnumber males five to one, presumably because of sexual differences in the shape of the acetabulum and the pelvis (Woolf and Turner, 1969; Simpson and Golbus, 1992). The recurrence risk for DDH in siblings is 4 percent for males and 8 percent for females, rising to 10–15 percent if a parent is also affected (Simpson and Golbus, 1992).

Traditional practices of infant care appear to significantly influence natural prevalence rates for DDH. Considerably higher rates are found in communities where infants are swaddled or diapered with their thighs extended, a position that separates the femur head from the acetabulum. Such practices are traditional in Japan, Turkey, and Saudi Arabia, as well as among Lapps and some Native American groups. A dramatic reduction in DDH prevalence occurred in a Japanese community when the traditional infant wrappings were abandoned (Yamamuro et al., 1984). Low rates of DDH occur in regions of Africa, China, and other communities where infants are carried on their mothers' backs with their thighs flexed and abducted (Salter, 1968). This position, which stabilizes the femoral head deep within the acetabulum, may correct many cases of congenital hip instability, preventing them from developing into dislocation (Edelson et al., 1984).

CONCLUSION

Birth defects impose a severe disease burden worldwide: they affect all major body systems and cause fetal deaths, neonatal and childhood deaths, and severe and lifelong disabilities. And for many birth defects, the stigma associated with the condition isolates affected individuals and their families and creates substantial social, psychological, and economic hardship.

The patterns of occurrence of birth defects in developing countries reveal a wide range of causes and risk factors for a wide range of conditions. In the absence of basic preventive public health measures, birth defects occur with increased frequency: Down syndrome where family planning services are deficient or underutilized; neural tube defects where periconceptional intake of folic acid is inadequate; iodine deficiency syndrome where iodized salt is not available; congenital rubella where populations are unvaccinated; cardiovascular and CNS damage where maternal control of insulin-dependent diabetes mellitus is poor; fetal alcohol syndrome where alcohol abuse occurs; and other birth defects where pregnant women are exposed to teratogenic drugs and pollutants.

Affordable, practical interventions are available to prevent some of the more common and severe birth defects. For populations where these particularly cost-effective interventions are being used effectively, there are additional cost-effective ways to further reduce the impact of birth defects through improved prevention and expanded treatment. To implement these interventions cost-effectively, policy makers need information about the occurrence of specific birth defects and risk factors in their populations, and the clinical- and cost-effectiveness of specific interventions.

REFERENCES

Adab N, Winterbottom J, Tudur C, Williamson PR. 2001. Common antiepileptic drugs in pregnancy in women with epilepsy. *Cochrane Database of Systematic Reviews* (2):1–14.

Akinyanju OO. 1989. A profile of sickle cell disease in Nigeria. *Annals of the New York Academy of Sciences* 565:126–136.

Alford CA, Pass RF. 1981. Epidemiology of chronic congenital and perinatal infections of man. *Clinics in Perinatology* 8(3):397–414.

Alford CA, Stagno S, Pass RF, Britt WJ. 1990. Congenital and perinatal cytomegalovirus infections. *Review of Infectious Diseases* 12(suppl 7):745–753.

Al-Gazali LI, Sztriha L, Dawodu A, Bakir M, Varghese M, Varady E, Scorer J, Abdulrazzaq YM, Bener A, Padmanabhan R. 1999. Pattern of central nervous system anomalies in a population with a high rate of consanguineous marriages. *Clinical Genetics* 55(2):95–102.

Ali O. 1995. Iodine deficiency disorders: A public health challenge in developing countries. *Nutrition* 11(5 suppl):517–520.

Ali ZA, Hull B, Lewis M. 1986. Neonatal manifestation of congenital rubella following an outbreak in Trinidad. *Journal of Tropical Pediatrics* 32(2):79–82.

Allison AC, Clyde DF. 1961. Malaria in African children with deficient erythrocyte glucose-6-phosphate dehydrogenase. *British Medical Journal* I:1346–1349.

Ang KC, Lee EH, Lee PY, Tan KL. 1997. An epidemiological study of developmental dysplasia of the hip in infants in Singapore. *Annals of the Academy of Medicine, Singapore* 26(4):456–458.

Angastiniotis M, Modell B, Englezos P, Boulyjenkov V. 1995. Prevention and control of haemoglobinopathies. *Bulletin of the World Health Organization* 73(3):375–386.

Annas GJ, Elias S. 1999. Thalidomide and the Titanic: Reconstructing the technology tragedies of the twentieth century. *American Journal of Public Health* 89(1):98–101.

Antia AU. 1974. Congenital heart disease in Nigeria. Clinical and necropsy study of 260 cases. *Archives of Disease in Childhood* 49(1):36–39.

Arpino C, Brescianini S, Robert E, Castilla EE, Cocchi G, Cornel MC, de Vigan C, Lancaster PA, Merlob P, Sumiyoshi Y, Zampino G, Renzi C, Rosano A, Mastroiacovo P. 2000. Teratogenic effects of antiepileptic drugs: Use of an international database on Malformations and Drug Exposure (MADRE). *Epilepsia* 41(11):1436–1443.

Ashley-Koch A, Yang Q, Olney RS. 2000. Sickle hemoglobin (Hb S) allele and sickle cell disease: A HuGE REVIEW. *American Journal of Epidemiology* 151(9):839–845.

Banatvala JE. 1998. Rubella—could do better. *Lancet* 351(9106):849–850.

Baxter DN. 1986. Control of the congenital rubella syndrome in Jamaica. *West Indian Medical Journal* 35(1):50–54.

Bellis G, Roux F, Chaventre A. 1998. Endemic cretinism in a traditional society in Mali: From the collectivity to the individual. *Collegium Antropologicum* 22(1):23–30.

Bello C, Whittle H. 1991. Cytomegalovirus infection in Gambian mothers and their babies. *Journal of Clinical Pathology* 44(5):366–369.

Bialik V, Bialik GM, Blazer S, Sujov P, Weiner F, Berant M. 1999. Developmental dysplasia of the hip: A new approach to incidence. *Pediatrics* 103(1):93–99.

Bittles AH, Mason WM, Greene J, Rao NA. 1991. Reproductive behavior and health in consanguineous marriages. *Science* 252(5007):789–794.

Bleichrodt N, Drenth PJ, Querido A. 1980. Effects of iodine deficiency on mental and psychomotor abilities. *American Journal of Physical Anthropology* 53(1):55–67.

Bos P, Steele D, Alexander J. 1995. Prevalence of antibodies to rubella, herpes simplex 2 and cytomegalovirus in pregnant women and in neonates at Ga-Rankuwa. *Central African Journal of Medicine* 41(1):14–17.

Boyages SC, Collins J, Jupp JJ, Morris J, Maberly GF, Eastman CJ. 1987. Congenital iodine deficiency disorders (endemic cretinism) history and description. *Australian and New Zealand Journal of Developmental Disabilities* 13:3–11.

Briggs GG, Freeman RK, Yaffe SJ. 1994. *Drugs in Pregnancy and Lactation.* 4th edition. Baltimore: Williams & Wilkins.

Brock DJH. 1996. Prenatal screening for cystic fibrosis: 5 years' experience reviewed. *Lancet* 347(8995):148–150.

Broor S, Kapil A, Kishore J, Seth P. 1991. Prevalence of rubella virus and cytomegalovirus infections in suspected cases of congenital infections. *Indian Journal of Pediatrics* 58(1): 75–78.

Brown ZA, Selke S, Zeh J, Kopelman J, Maslow A, Ashley RL, Watts DH, Berry S, Herd M, Corey L. 1997. The acquisition of herpes simplex virus during pregnancy. *New England Journal of Medicine* 337(8):509–515.

Carey L, Handsfield HH. 2000. Genital herpes and public health: Addressing a global problem. *Journal of the American Medical Association* 283(6):791–794.

Carothers AD, Castilla EE, Dutra MG, Hook EB. 2001. Search for ethnic, geographic and other factors in the epidemiology of Down syndrome in South America: Analysis of data from the ECLAMC project, 1967–1997. *American Journal of Medical Genetics* 103(2):149–156.

Cartmill TB, DuShane JW, McGoon DC, Kirklin JW. 1966. Results of repair of ventricular septal defect. *Journal of Thoracic and Cardiovascular Surgery* 52(4):486–501.

Castilla EE, Lopez-Camelo JS. 1990. The surveillance of birth defects in South America: I. The search for time clusters: Epidemics. *Advances in Mutagenesis Research* 2:191–210.

Castilla EE, Sod R. 1990. The surveillance of birth defects in South America: II. The search for geographic clusters. *Advances in Mutagenesis Research* 2:211–230.

Castilla EE, Gomez MA, Lopez-Camelo J, Paz JE. 1991. Frequency of first-cousin marriages from civil marriage certificates in Argentina. *Human Biology* 63(2):203–210.

Castilla EE, Ashton-Prolla P, Barreda-Mejia E, Brunoni D, Cavalcanti DP, Correa-Neto J, Delgadillo JL, Dutra MG, Felix T, Giraldo A, Juarez N, Lopez-Camelo JS, Nazer J, Orioli IM, Paz JE, Pessoto MA, Pina-Neto JM, Quadrelli R, Rittler M, Rueda S, Saltos M, Sanchez O, Schuler L. 1996. Thalidomide, a current teratogen in South America. *Teratology* 54(6):273–277.

Castilla EE, Rittler M, Dutra MG, Lopez-Camelo JS, Campana H, Paz JE, Orioli IM. 1998. Survival of children with Down syndrome in South America. ECLAMC-Down survey Group. Latin American Collaborative Study of Congenital Malformations. *American Journal of Medical Genetics* 79(2):108–111.

Chambers CD, Johnson KA, Dick LM, Felix RJ, Jones KL. 1998. Maternal fever and birth outcome: A prospective study. *Teratology* 58(6):251–257.

Chaturvedi UC, Tripathi BN, Mathur A, Singh UK, Mehrotra RM. 1976. Role of rubella in congenital malformations in India. *Journal of Hygiene* 76(1):33–40.

Chintana T. 1991. Pattern of antibodies in toxoplasmosis of pregnant women and their children in Thailand. *Southeast Asian Journal of Tropical Medicine and Public Health* 22(suppl):107–110.

Choudhury AR, Mukherjee M, Sharma A, Talukder G, Ghosh PK. 1989. Study of 1,26,266 consecutive births for major congenital defects. *Indian Journal of Pediatrics* 56(4):493–499.

Christianson AL. 1996. Down syndrome in sub-Saharan Africa. *Journal of Medical Genetics* 33(2):89–92.

Christianson AL, Venter PA, Modiba JH., Nelson MM. 2000. Development of a primary health care clinical genetic service in rural South Africa—the Northern Province experience, 1990–1996.*Community Genetics* 3(2):77–84.

Chuangsuwanich A, Aojanepong C, Muangsombut S, Tongpiew P. 1998. Epidemiology of cleft lip and palate in Thailand. *Annals of Plastic Surgery* 41(1):7–10.

Coelho KE, Sarmento MF, Veiga CM, Speck-Martins CE, Safatle HP, Castro CV, Niikawa N. 2000. Misoprostol embryotoxicity: Clinical evaluation of fifteen patients with arthrogryposis. *American Journal of Medical Genetics* 95(4):297–301.

Cohen AJ, Tamir A, Houri S, Abegaz B, Gilad E, Omohkdion S, Zabeeda D, Khazin V, Ciubotaru A, Schachner A. 2001. Save a child's heart: We can and we should. *Annals of Thoracic Surgery* 71(2):407–408.

Cook AJ, Gilbert RE, Buffolano W, Zufferey J, Petersen E, Jenum PA, Foulon W, Semprini AE, Dunn DT. 2000. Sources of toxoplasma infection in pregnant women: European multicentre case-control study. *British Medical Journal* 321(7254):142–147.

Cooper ME, Stone RA, Liu Y, Hu DN, Melnick M, Marazita ML. 2000. Descriptive epidemiology of nonsyndromic cleft lip with or without cleft palate in Shanghai, China, from 1980 to 1989. *Cleft Palate-Craniofacial Journal* 37(3):274–280.

Croen LA, Shaw GM. 1995. Young maternal age and congenital malformations: A population-based study. *American Journal of Public Health* 85(5):710–713.

Croxford J, Viljoen D. 1999. Alcohol consumption by pregnant women in the Western Cape. *South African Medical Journal* 89(9):962–965.

Cunningham G. 2000. Phenyletonuria and other inherited metabolic defects. In Wald N, Leck I (eds.). *Antenatal and Neonatal Screening,* 2nd edition. Oxford, UK: Oxford University Press. P. 353.

Cutts FT, Vynnycky E. 1999. Modelling the incidence of congenital rubella syndrome in developing countries. *International Journal of Epidemiology* 28(6):1176–1184.

Cutts FT, Robertson SE, Diaz-Ortega JL, Samuel R. 1997. Control of rubella and congenital rubella syndrome (CRS) in developing countries, Part 1. Burden of disease from CRS. *Bulletin of the World Health Organization* 75(1):55–68.

Czeizel AE, Dudas I. 1992. Prevention of the first occurrence of neural-tube defects by periconceptional vitamin supplementation. *New England Journal of Medicine* 327(26): 1832–1835.

DeLong GR, Stanbury JB, Fierro-Benitez R. 1985. Neurological signs in congenital iodine-deficiency disorder (endemic cretinism). *Developmental Medicine and Child Neurology* 27(3):317–324.

Dietz FR. 1985. On the pathogenesis of clubfoot. *Lancet* 1(8425):388–390.

Diggle GE. 2001. Thalidomide: 40 years on. *International Journal of Clinical Practice* 55(9): 627–631.

Doehring E, Reiter-owona I, Bauer O, Kaisi M, Hlobil H, Quade G, Hamudu NA, Seitz HM. 1995. *Toxoplasma gondii* antibodies in pregnant women and their newborns in Dar es Salaam, Tanzania. *American Journal of Tropical Medical Hygiene* 52(6):546–548.

Doraisingham S, Goh KT. 1981. The rubella immunity of women of child-bearing age in Singapore. *Annals of the Academy of Medicine Singapore* 10(2):238–241.

Dowdle WR, Ferrera W, De Salles Gomes LF, King D, Kourany M, Madalengoitia J, Pearson E, Swanston WH, Tosi HC, Vilches AM. 1970. WHO collaborative study on the sero-epidemiology of rubella in Caribbean and Middle and South American populations in 1968. *Bulletin of the World Health Organization* 42(3):419–422.

Dubey JP. 2000. Sources of *Toxoplama gondii* infection in pregnancy: Until rates of congenital toxoplasmosis fall, control measures are essential. *British Medical Journal* 321(7254): 127–128.

Dunn JT. 1994. Societal implications of iodine deficiency and the value of its prevention. In Stanbury, JB (ed.). *The Damaged Brain of Iodine Deficiency*. New York: Cognizant Communications. Pp. 309–314.

Dunn PM, Evans RE, Thearle MJ, Griffiths HED, Witherow PJ. 1985. Congenital dislocation of the hip: Early and late diagnosis and management compared. *Archives of Diseases in Children* 60:607–614.

Durkin MS, Hasan ZM, Hasan KZ. 1998. Prevalence and correlates of mental retardation among children in Karachi, Pakistan. *American Journal of Epidemiology* 147(3):281–288.

ECLAMC (Latin American Collaborative Study of Congenital Malformations). 2001. Available online at http://www.eclamcnet.net.

Edelson JG, Hirsch M, Weinberg H, Attar D, Barmeir E. 1984. Congential dislocation of the hip and computerised axial tomography. *Journal of Bone and Joint Surgery* 66(4):472–478.

Eisensmith RC, Woo SL. 1994. Population genetics of phenylketonuria. *Acta Paediatrica* 407(suppl):19–26.

Elango S, Reddy TNK, Shriwas SR. 1994. Ocular abnormalities in children from Malaysian school for the deaf. *Annals of Tropical Pediatrics* 14(2):149–152.

El-Hazmi MA, Warsy AS. 1996. Genetic disorders among Arab populations. *Saudi Medical Journal* 17(2):108–123.

Essawy M, Khashaba A, Magda A, el-Kholy M, Elmeya S, Samy G. 1990. Study of congenital toxoplasmosis in Egyptian newborns. *Journal of Egyptian Public Health Association* 65(5–6):669–680.

Expanded Programme on Immunization. Rubella outbreak, Oman. *Weekly Epidemiological Record* 69(45):333–336.

Fattibene P, Mazzei F, Nuccetelli C, Risica S. 1999. Prenatal exposure to ionizing radiation: Sources, effects and regulatory aspects. *Acta Paediatrica* 88(7):693–702.

Fauci AS, Eugene B, Isselbacher KJ, Wilson JD, Martin JB, Kasper DL, Hauser SL, Longo DL (eds.). 2001. *Harrison's Principles of Internal Medicine*, 14th edition. Vol. 2. New York: McGraw-Hill. Pp. 649, 651.

Fenig E, Mishaeli M, Kalish Y, Lishner M. 2001. Pregnancy and radiation. *Cancer Treatment Reviews* 27(1):1–7.

Finelli L, Berman SM, Koumans EH, Levine WC. 1998. Congenital syphilis. *Bulletin of the World Health Organization* 76(suppl 2):126–128.

Fogel A, Gerichter CB, Rannon L, Bernholtz B, Handsher R. 1976. Serologic studies in 11,460 pregnant women during the 1972 rubella epidemic in Israel. *American Journal of Epidemiology* 103(1):51–59.

Fowler KB, Stagno S, Pass RF, Britt WJ, Bott TJ, Alford CA. 1992. The outcome of congenital cytomegalovirus infection in relation to maternal antibody status. *New England Journal of Medicine* 326(10):663–667.

Friberg L, et al. (Expert Group, National Institute of Public Health, Stockholm). 1971. Methylmercury in fish: A toxicologic–epidemiologic evaluation of risks. *Nordisk hygienisk tidskrift* 4(suppl):19–364.

Gandahusada S. 1991. Study on the prevalence of toxoplasmosis in Indonesia: A review. *Southeast Asian Journal of Tropical Medicine and Public Health* 22(suppl): 93–98.

Geelhoed GW. 1999. Metabolic maladaptation: Individual and social consequences of medical intervention in correcting endemic hypothyroidism. *Nutrition* 15(11–12):908–932; discussion 939.

Ghebrekidan H, Ruden U, Cox S, Wahren B, Grandien M. 1999. Prevalence of herpes simplex virus types 1 and 2, cytomegalovirus, and varicella-zoster virus infections in Eritrea. *Journal of Clinical Virology* 12(1):53–64.

Gonzalez CH, Marques-Dias MJ, Kim CA, Da Paz JA, Huson SM, Holmes LB. 1998. Congenital abnormalities in Brazilian children associated with misoprostol misuse in first trimester of pregnancy. *Lancet* 351(9116):1624–1627.

Graham JM Jr., Edwards MJ, Edwards MJ. 1998. Teratogen update: Gestational effects of maternal hyperthermia due to febrile illnesses and resultant patterns of defects in humans. *Teratology* 58(5):209–211.

Granda H, Gispert S, Dorticos A, Martin M, Cuadras Y, Calvo M, Martinez G, Zayas MA, Oliva JA, Heredero L. 1991. Cuban programme for prevention of sickle cell disease. *Lancet* 337(8734):152–153.

Granda H, Gispert S, Martinez G, Gomez M, Ferreira R, Collazo T, Magarino C, Heredero L. 1994. Results from a reference laboratory for prenatal diagnosis of sickle cell disorders in Cuba. *Prenatal Diagnosis* 14(8):659–662.

Grody WW, Cutting GR, Klinger KW, Richards CS, Watson MS, Desnick RJ. 2001. Laboratory standards and guidelines for population-based cystic fibrosis carrier screening. *Genetics in Medicine* 3(2):149–154.

Gross RH, Cox A, Tatyrek R, Pollay M, Barnes WA. 1983. Early management and decision making for the treatment of myelomeningocele. *Pediatrics* 72(4):450–458.

Grover JK, Vats V, Gopalakrishna R, Ramam M. 2000. Thalidomide: A re-look. *National Medical Journal of India* 13(3):132–141.

Gunasekera DP, Gunaserkera PC. 1996. Rubella immunisation—learning from developed countries. *Lancet* 347(9016):1694–1695.

Gurson CT, Sertel H, Gurkan M, Pala S. 1973. Newborn screening for cystic fibrosis with the chloride electrode and neutron activation analysis. *Helvetica Paediatrica Acta* 28(2):165–174.

Halpern JP, Boyages SC, Maberly GF, Eastman CJ, Collins JK, Morris JGL. 1991. The neurology of endemic cretinism: A study of two endemias. *Brain* 114(Pt 2):825–841.

Handin RI. 1998. Disorders of coagulation and thrombosis. In Fauci A, Braunwald E, Isslebacher KJ, Wilson JD, Martin JB, Kasper DL, Hauser SL, Longo DL (eds.). *Harrison's Principles of Internal Medicine*, 14th edition. New York: Mc-Graw Hill. Pp. 736–743.

Hanshaw JB, Dudgeon JA, Marshall WC. 1985. *Viral Diseases of the Fetus and Newborn,* 2nd edition. Vol. 17 of Major Problems in Clinical Pediatrics. Philadelphia: W.B. Saunders Co. P. 3.

Hardman J, Goodman A, Gilman L, Limbird L. 1996. *Goodman and Gilman's: The Pharmacological Basis of Therapeutics,* 9th edition. New York: McGraw-Hill Professional.

Herring JA. 1990. Congenital dislocation of the hip. In Morrissy RT (ed.). *Lovell and Winter's Pediatric Orthopaedics,* 3rd edition. Philadelphia: J.B. Lippincott. Pp. 815–830.

Hizel S, Parker S, Onde U. 1999. Seroprevalence of cytomegalovirus infection among children and females in Ankara, Turkey, 1995. *Pediatrics International* 41(5):506–509.

Hoffman JI, Kaplan S. 2002. The incidence of congenital heart disease. *Journal of the American College of Cardiology* 39(12):1890–1900.

Hollowell JG Jr., Hannon WH. 1997. Teratogen update: Iodine deficiency, a community teratogen. *Teratology* 55(6):389–405.

Holmes LB, Harvey EA, Coull BA, Huntington KB, Khosibin S, Hayes AM, Ryan LM. 2001. The teratogenicity of anticonvulsant drugs. *New England Journal of Medicine* 344(15): 1132–1138.

Hook EB. 1981. Rates of chromosome abnormalities at different maternal ages. *Obstetrics and Gynecology* 58(3):282–285.

Hook EB. 1982. The epidemiology of Down syndrome. In Pueschel SM (ed.). *Down Syndrome: Advances in Biomedicine and the Behavioral Sciences.* Cambridge, MA: Ware Press. Pp. 11–18.

Hook EB. 1992. Prevalence, risk, and recurrence. In Brock DJH, Rodeck CH, Ferguson-Smith MA (eds.). *Prenatal Diagnosis and Screening.* Edinburgh: Churchill Livingstone. Pp. 351–392.

Hunt GM. 1990. Open spina bifida: Outcome for a complete cohort treated unselectively and followed into adulthood. *Developmental Medicine and Child Neurology* 32(2):108–118.

Hussain R, Bittles AH. 1998. The prevalence and demographic characteristics of consanguineous marriages in Pakistan. *Journal of Biosocial Science* 30(2):261–275.

Institute of Medicine (IOM). 1996. Stratton K, Howe C, Battaglia F (eds.). *Fetal Alcohol Syndrome: Diagnosis, Epidemiology, Prevention, and Treatment.* Washington, DC: National Academy Press.

Institute of Medicine (IOM). 2000. *Toxicological Effects of Methylmercury.* Washington, DC: National Academy Press. P. 344.

Institute of Medicine (IOM). 2003. *Improving Birth Outcomes: Meeting the Challenge in the Developing World.* Washington, DC: The National Academies Press.

International Clearinghouse for Birth Defects Monitoring Systems. 2001. Available online at http://www.icbd.org/publications.htm#WorldAtlasofBirthDefects.

Jaber L, Merlob P, Bu X, Rotter JI, Shohat M. 1992. Marked parental consanguinity as a cause for increased major malformations in an Israeli Arab community. *American Journal of Medical Genetics* 44(1):1–6.

Jacobson JL, Jacobson SW. 1996. Intellectual impairment in children exposed to polychlorinated biphenyls in utero. *New England Journal of Medicine* 335(11):783–789.

Jalil MQ, Mia MJ, Ali SM. 1997. Epidemiological study of endemic cretinism in a hyperendemic area. *Bangladesh Medical Research Council Bulletin* 23(1):34–37.

Kale JS. 1999. Haemophilia: Scope for rehabilitation in India. *Journal of Postgraduate Medicine* 45(4):126.

Kalter H, Warkany J. 1983. (Medical Progress) Congenital malformations etiologic factors and their role in prevention. *New England Journal of Medicine* 308(8):424–431(Part I); 491–497(Part II).

Kaur R, Gupta N, Nair D, Kakkar M, Mathur MD. 1999. Screening for TORCH infections in pregnant women: A report from Delhi. *Southeast Asian Journal of Tropical Medicine and Public Health* 30(2):284–286.

Keeler C. 1970. Cuna moon-child albinism, 1950–1970. *Journal of Heredity* 61(6):273–278.

Khare S, Banerjee K, Padubidri V, Rai A, Kumari S, Kumari S. 1987. Lowered immunity status of rubella virus infection in pregnant women. *Journal of Communicable Diseases* 19(4):391–395.

Khare S, Gupta HL, Banerjee K, Kumari S, Kumari S, Gupta HL. 1990. Seroimmunity to rubella virus infection in young adult females in Delhi. *Journal of Communicable Diseases* 22(4):279–280.

Khlat M, Khoury M. 1991. Inbreeding and diseases: Demographic, genetic, and epidemiologic perspectives. *Epidemiology Review* 13:28–41.

Khlat M, Teebi AS, Farag TI (eds.). 1997. *Endogamy in the Arab World*. New York: Oxford University Press.

Khoury MJ, Becerra JE, Cordero JF, Erickson JD. 1989. Clinical-epidemiologic assessment of pattern of birth defects associated with human teratogens: Application to diabetic embryopathy. *Pediatrics* 84(4):658–665.

Kietduriyakul V, Leangphibul P, Tongkittikul K. 1988. Study of phenylketonuria in Thai children. *Journal of the Medical Association of Thailand* 71(5):258–261.

Kirklin JW, Barrat-Boyes BG (eds.). 1993. Coarctation of the aorta, and interrupted aortic arch. *Cardiac Surgery,* 2nd edition. Vol. 2. New York: Churchill Livingstone. P. 1274.

Koren G (ed.). 1998. *Maternal-Fetal Toxicology: A Clinician's Guide,* 2nd edition. New York: Marcel Dekker. Pp. 115–128.

Koren G, Pastuszak A, Ito S. 1998. Drugs in pregnancy. *New England Journal of Medicine* 338(16):1126–1137.

Kouame P, Bellis G, Tebbi A, Gaimard M, Dilumbu I, Assouan A, Roux F, Mayer G, Chastin I, Diarra N, Chaventre A. 1998. The prevalence of goitre and cretinism in a population of the west Ivory Coast. *Collegium Antropologicum* 22(1):31–41.

Kromberg JG, Jenkins T. 1982. Prevalence of albinism in the South African negro. *South African Medical Journal* 61(11):383–386.

Kuliev AM, Modell B. 1990. Problems in the control of genetic disorders. *Biomedical Science* 1(1):3–17.

Kulkarni ML, Kurian M. 1990. Consanguinity and its effect on fetal growth and development: A south Indian study. *Journal of Medical Genetics* 27(6):348–352.

Lam SK. 1972. The seroepidemiology of rubella in Kuala Lumpur, West Malaysia. *Bulletin of the World Health Organization* 47(1):127–129.

Laurence KM. 1974. Effects of early surgery for spina bifida cystica on survival and quality of life. *Lancet* 1(7852):301–304.

Lawn JE, Reef S, Baffoe-Bonnie B, Adadevoh S, Caul EO, Griffin GE. 2000. Unseen blindness, unheard deafness, and unrecorded death and disability: Congenital rubella in Kumasi, Ghana. *American Journal of Public Health* 90(10):1555–1561.

Leck I. 1994. Structural birth defects. In Pless IB (ed.). *The Epidemiology of Childhood Disorders*. New York: Oxford University Press. Pp. 66–117.

Leck I. 2000. Congenital dislocation of the hip. In Wald N, Leck I (eds.). 2000. *Antenatal and Neonatal Screening,* 2nd edition. New York: Oxford University Press. Pp. 398–424.

Liascovich R, Castilla EE, Rittler M. 2001. Consanguinity in South America: Demographic aspects. *Human Heredity* 51(1–2):27–34.

Loffredo CA, Wilson PD, Ferencz C. 2001. Maternal diabetes: An independent risk factor for major cardiovascular malformations with increased mortality of affected infants. *Teratology* 64(2):98–106.

Luande J, Henschke CI, Mohammed N. 1985. The Tanzanian human albino skin. Natural history. *Cancer* 55(8):1823–1828.

Lund PM. 1996. Distribution of oculocutaneous albinism in Zimbabwe. *Journal of Medical Genetics* 33(8):641–644.

Maberly GF. 1998. Iodine deficiency. *Bulletin of the World Health Organization* 76(suppl 2):118–120.

Maberly GF, Eastman CJ. 1976. Endemic goiter in Sarawak, Malaysia: I. Somatic growth and aetiology. *Southeast Asian Journal of Tropical Medicine and Public Health* 7(3):434–442.

Magenis RE, Hecht R, Mulham S Jr. 1968. Trisomy 13(D) syndrome: Studies on parental age, sex, ratio and survival. *Journal of Pediatrics* 73(2):222–228.

Manjunath N, Balaya S. 1984. Serological study on congenital rubella in Delhi. *Indian Journal of Medical Research* 79:716–721.

Marsh DO, Clarkson TW, Cox C, Myers GJ, Amin-Zaki L, Al-Tikriti S. 1987. Fetal methylmercury poisoning. Relationship between concentration in single strands of maternal hair and child effects. *Archives Suisses de Neurologie, Neurochirurgie et de Psychiatrie* 44(10):1017–1022.

Mathur A, Chaturvedi UC, Mehrotra RML. 1974. Serological study for the prevalence of rubella Lucknow. *Indian Journal of Medical Research* 62(2):307–312.

Mathur A, Tripathi R, Chaturvedi UC, Mehra P. 1982. Congenital rubella following inapparent rubella infection. *Indian Journal of Medical Research* 75:469–473.

May PA, Brooke L, Gossage JP, Croxford J, Adnams C, Jones KL, Robinson L, Viljoen D. 2000. Epidemiology of fetal alcohol syndrome in a South African community in the Western Cape Province. *American Journal of Public Health* 90(12):1905–1912.

McDonald AD, McDonald JC, Armstrong B, Cherry NM, Nolin AD, Robert D. 1989. Fathers' occupation and pregnancy outcome. *British Journal of Indian Medicine* 46(5):329–333.

McLaughlin JF, Shurtleff DB, Lamers JY, Stuntz JT, Hayden PW, Kropp RJ. 1985. Influence of prognosis on decisions regarding the care of newborns with myelodysplasia. *New England Journal of* Medicine 312(25):1589–1594.

Mendis L. 1989. Susceptibility to rubella virus among Lankan women. *Ceylon Medical Journal* 34(2):73–75.

Mittal M, Tandon M, Raghuvanshi RS. 2000. Iodine status of children and use of iodized salt in Tarai region of North India. *Journal of Tropical Pediatrics* 46(5):300–302.

Mokhtar MM, Kotb SM, Ismail SR. 1998. Autosomal recessive disorders among patients attending the genetics clinic in Alexandria. *Eastern Mediterranean Health Journal* 4(3):470–479.

MRC (Medical Research Council) Vitamin Study Research Group. 1991. Prevention of neural tube defects: Results of the Medical Research Council Vitamin Study. *Lancet* 338(8760):131–137.

Murray CJL, Lopez AD (eds.). 1996. *Health Dimensions of Sex and Reproduction: The Global Burden of Disease: A Comprehensive Assessment of Mortality and Disability from Diseases, Injuries, and Risk Factors in 1990 and Projected to 2020.* Boston: Harvard School of Public Health: Global Burden of Disease and Injury Series.

Murray CJ, Lopez AD (eds.). 1998. *Health Dimensions of Sex and Reproduction: The Global Burden of Sexually Transmitted Diseases, HIV, Maternal Conditions, Perinatal Disorders, and Congenital Anomalies.* Boston: Harvard School of Public Health: Global Burden of Disease and Injury Series.

Murshid WR. 2000. Spina bifida in Saudi Arabia: Is consanguinity among the parents a risk factor? *Pediatric Neurosurgery* 32(1):10–12.

Nadeem RD, Brown JK, Lawson G, Mcnicol MF. 2000. Somatosensory evoked potentials as a means of assessing neurological abnormality in congenital talipes equinovarus. *Developmental Medicine and Child Neurology* 42(8):525–530.

Nahmias AJ, Lee FK, Beckman-Nahmias S. 1990. Sero-epidemiological and -sociological patterns of herpes simplex virus infection in the world. *Scandinavian Journal of Infectious Diseases* 69(suppl):19–36.

Nazer HM. 1992. Early diagnosis of cystic fibrosis in Jordanian children. *Journal of Tropical Pediatrics* 38(3):113–115.

Nicolaidis P, Petersen MB. 1998. Origin and review of non-disjunction in human autosomal trisomies. *Human Reproduction* 13(2):313–319.

Oberle MW, Rosero-Bixby L, Lee FK, Sanchez-Braverman M, Nahmias AJ, Guinan ME. 1989. Herpes simplex virus type 2 antibodies: High prevalence in monogamous women in Costa Rica. *American Journal of Tropical Medicine and Hygiene* 41(2):224–229.

Odelola HA. 1978. Rubella haemagglutination-inhibiting antibodies in females of child-bearing age in Western Nigeria. *Journal of Hygiene, Epidemiology, Microbiology and Immunology* 22(2):190–194.

O'Farrell N. 1999. Increasing prevalence of genital herpes in developing countries: Implications for heterosexual HIV transmission and STI control programmes. *Sexually Transmitted Infections* 75(6):377–384.

Okoro AN. 1975. Albinism in Nigeria. A clinical and social study. *British Journal of Dermatology* 92(5):485–492.

Olshan AF, Teschke K, Baird PA. 1990. Birth defects among offspring of firemen. *American Journal of Epidemiology* 131(2):312–321.

Onadeko MO, Joynson DH, Payne RA, Francis J. 1996. The prevalence of toxoplasma antibodies in pregnant Nigerian women and the occurrence of stillbirth and congenital malformation. *African Journal of Medicine and Medical Sciences* 25(4):331–334.

Online Mendelian Inheritance in Man (OMIM). 2002. Available online at http://www.ncbi.nlm.nih.gov/Omim/. National Center for Biotechnology Information: Johns Hopkins.

Orioli IM, Castilla EE. 2000. Epidemiological assessment of misoprostol teratogenicity. *BJOG: An International Journal of Obstetrics and Gynaecology* 107(4):519–523.

Owens CS, Espino RT. 1989. Rubella in Panama: Still a problem. *Pediatric Infectious Disease Journal* 8:110–115.

Ozalp I, Coskun T, Tokol S, Demircin G, Monch E. 1990. Inherited metabolic disorders in Turkey. *Journal of Inherited Metabolic Disorders* 13(5):732–738.

Padoa C, Goldman A, Jenkins T, Ramsay M. 1999. Cystic fibrosis carrier frequencies in populations of African origin. *Journal of Medical Genetics* 36(1):41–44.

Penchaszadeh VB. 1994. Genetics and public health. *Bulletin of the Pan American Health Organization* 28(1):62–72.

Phiromsawat S, Tongyai T, O-Prasertsawat P, Kanachareon A, Imsoon L, Bhodipala P, Chaturachinda K. 1988. Rubella: A serologic study in pregnant women at Ramathibodi Hospital (1984–1985) *Journal of the Medical Association of Thailand* 71(suppl 2):26–28.

Platt LD, Koch R, Hanley WB, Levy HL, Matalon R, Rouse B, Trefz F, de la Cruz F, Guttler F, Azen C, Friedman EG. 2000. The international study of pregnancy outcome in women with maternal phenylketonuria: Report of a 12-year study. *American Journal of Obstetrics and Gynecology* 2(2):326–333.

Polifka JE, Friedman JM. 1999. Clinical teratology: Identifying teratogenic risks in humans. *Clinical Genetics* 56(6):409–420.

Polifka JE, Dolan CR, Donlan MA, Friedman JM. 1996. Clinical teratology counseling and consultation report: High dose beta-carotene use during early pregnancy. *Teratology* 54(2):103–107.

Pruksananonda P, Bumrungtrakul P. 1983. Serosurvey of rubella antibody among health personnel of Songklanagarind University Hospital. Thailand. *Southeast Asian Journal of Tropical Medicine and Public Health* 14(3):380–384.

Ramsay MC, Reynolds CR. 2000. Does smoking by pregnant women influence IQ, birth weight, and developmental disabilities in their infants? A methodological review and multivariate analysis. *Neuropsychology Review* 10(1):1–40.

Roth EF, Raventos-Suarez C, Rinaldi A, Nagel RL. 1983. Glucose-6-phosphate dehydrogenase deficiency inhibits in vitro growth of *Plasmodium falciparum*. *Proceedings of the National Academy of Sciences* 80(1):298–299.

Rygg IH, Olesen K, Boesen I. 1971. The life history of tetralogy of Fallot. *Danish Medical Bulletin* 18(suppl 2):25–30.

Salisbury DM, Savinykh AI. 1991. Rubella and congenital rubella syndrome in developing countries. Document EPI/GAG/91/WP.15. Presented at the Global Advisory Group Meeting, Antalya, Turkey, October 14–18.

Salter RB. 1968. Etiology, pathogenesis and possible prevention of congenital dislocation of the hip. *Canadian Medical Association Journal* 98(20):933–945.

Salzano FM. 1985. Incidence, effects, and management of sickle cell disease in Brazil. *American Journal of Pediatric Hematology and Oncology* 7(3):240–244.

Sampson PD, Streissguth AP, Bookstein FL, Little RE, Clarren SK, Dehaene P, Hanson JW, Graham JM Jr. 1997. Incidence of fetal alcohol syndrome and prevalence of alcohol-related neurodevelopmental disorder. *Teratology* 56(5):317–326.

Samren EB, van Duijn CM, Christiaens GC, Hofman A, Lindhout D. 1999. Antiepileptic drug regimens and major congenital abnormalities in the offspring. *Annals of Neurology* 46(5):739–746.

Sankar R, Pulger T, Rai B, Gomathi S, Gyatso TR, Pandav CS. 1998. Epidemiology of endemic cretinism in Sikkim, India. *Indian Journal of Pediatrics* 65(2):303–309.

Satpathy G. 1989. Seroepidemiology of rubella in Indian women and in children with congenital malformations. *Virus Information Exchange Newsletter* 6(3):126.

Schull WJ, Otake M. 1999. Cognitive function and perinatal exposure to ionizing radiation. *Teratology* 59(4):222–226.

Scriver CR, Clow CL. 1980. Phenylketonuria: Epitome of human biochemical genetics (first of two parts). *New England Journal of Medicine* 303(23):1396.

Shibuya K, Murray C. 1998. Congenital anomalies. In Murray C, Lopez A (eds.). 1998. *Health Dimensions of Sex and Reproduction*. Boston: Harvard School of Public Health. Pp. 463, 466–467, 470, 473.

Simpson JL, Golbus MS. 1992. *Genetics in Obstetrics and Gynecology*, 2nd edition. Philadelphia: W.B. Saunders Co. Pp. 61–78, 87, 92, 133–163.

Sinha SN. 1987. A simple guide to management of club foot. *Papua New Guinea Medical Journal* 30(2):165–168.

Smith JB, Burton NF, Nelson G, Fortney JA, Duale S. 1986. Hospital deaths in a high risk obstetric population: Karawa, Zaire. *International Journal of Gynaecology and Obstetrics* 24(3):225–234.

Smith J, Taddio KA, Koren G. 1994. Drugs of choice for pregnant women. In Koren G (ed.). *Maternal-Fetal Toxicology: A Clinician's Guide,* 2nd edition. New York: Marcel Dekker. Pp. 115–128.

Sohn YM, Park KI, Lee C, Han DG, Lee WY. 1992. Congenital cytomegalovirus infection in Korean population with very high prevalence of maternal immunity. *Journal of Korean Medical Science* 7(1):47–51.

Stagno S, Whitley RJ. 1985. Herpes virus infections of pregnancy. Part I. Cytomegalovirus and Epstein-Barr virus infections. *New England Journal of Medicine* 13(20):1270–1274.

Stagno S, Pass RF, Dworsky ME, Alford CA Jr. 1982. Maternal cytomegalovirus infection and perinatal transmission. *Clinical Obstetrics and Gynecology* 25(3):563–576.

Stagno S, Pass RF, Dworsky ME, Alford CA. 1984. Congenital and perinatal cytomegalovirus infections. In Amstey MS (ed.). *Virus Infections in Pregnancy.* New York: Grune and Stratton. Pp. 105–123.

Stanbury JB (ed.). 1994. *The Damaged Brain of Iodine Deficiency: Cognitive, Behavioral, Neuromotor, Educative Aspects.* New York: Cognizant Communication Corporation.

Steensma DP, Hoyer JD, Fairbanks VF. 2001. Hereditary red blood cell disorders in Middle Eastern patients. *Mayo Clinic Proceedings* 76(3):285–293.

St. John MA, Benjamin S. 2000. An epidemic of congenital rubella in Barbados. *Annals of Tropical Paediatrics* 20(3):231–235.

Sweeting I, Serjeant BE, Serjeant GR, Kulozik AE, Vetter B, 1998. HB S–HB Monroe: A sickle cell–beta-thalassemia syndrome. *Hemoglobin* 22(2):153–156.

Taechowisan T, Sutthent R, Louisirirotchanskul S, Puthavathana P, Wasi C. 1997. Immune status in congenital infections by TORCH agents in pregnant Thais. *Asian Pacific Journal of Allergy and Immunology* 15(2):93–97.

Tan KL, Wong TT, Chan MC, Chun FY, Lam SK. 1970. Congenital rubella in Singapore. *Journal of the Singapore Paediatric Society* 12(2):111–125.

Tantivanich S, Savanat T, Vongsthongsri U, Manesuwan P. 1980. Serological studies on possible causes of intra-uterine infections in Thai infants. *Southeast Asian Journal of Tropical Medicine and Public Health* 11(3):387–394.

United Nations Children's Fund (UNICEF). 1998. *The State of the World's Children 1999.* New York: UNICEF.

Vanchieri C. 1997. Preparing for thalidomide's comeback. *Annals of Internal Medicine* 127(10):951–952.

van der Put NM, Gabreels F, Stevens EM, Smeitink JA, Trijbels FJ, Eskes TK, van den Heuvel LP, Blom HJ. 1998. A second common mutation in the methylenetetrahydrofolate reductase gene: An additional risk factor for neural-tube defects? *American Journal of Human Genetics* 62(5):1044–1051.

Vargas FR, Schuler-Faccini L, Brunoni D, Kim C, Meloni VF, Sugayama SM, Albano L, Llerena JC Jr., Almeida JC, Duarte A, Cavalcanti DP, Goloni-Bertollo E, Conte A, Koren G, Addis A. 2000. Prenatal exposure to misoprostol and vascular disruption defects: A case-control study. *American Journal of Medical Genetics* 95(4):302–306.

Verjee ZH. 1993. Glucose 6-phosphate dehydrogenase deficiency in Africa—review. *East African Medical Journal* 70(4 suppl):40–47.

Viljoen D. 1999. Fetal alcohol syndrome. *South African Medical Journal* 89(9):958–960.

Viljoen D, Craig P. 2001. *Epidemiological Studies for Fetal Alcohol Syndrome in Four Gauteng Communities.* Report to the National Department of Health, Directorate Mental Health and Substance Abuse, Pretoria.

Viljoen DL, Carr LG, Foroud TM, Brooke L, Ramsay M, Li TK. 2001. Alcohol dehydrogenase-2*2 allele is associated with decreased prevalence of fetal alcohol syndrome in the mixed-ancestry population of the Western Cape Province, South Africa. *Alcoholism, Clinical and Experimental Research* 25(12):1719–1722.

Warkany J. 1986. Teratogen update: Hyperthermia. *Teratology* 33(3):365–371.

Weatherall DJ. 1997. The thalassemias. *British Medical Journal* 314(7095):1675–1678.

Weatherall DJ, Clegg JB. 2001. Inherited hemoglobin disorders: An increasing global health problem. *Bulletin of the World Health Organization* 79(8):704–712.

Whitley RJ, Arvin A, Prober C, Burchett S, Corey L, Powell D, Plotkin S, Starr S, Alfodd C, Connor J, Jacobs RF, Nahmias AJ, Soong, SJ. 1991. A controlled trial comparing vidarabine with acyclovir in neonatal herpes simplex virus infection. Infectious Diseases Collaborative Antiviral Study Group. *New England Journal of Medicine* 324(4):444–449.

Wilcken DE. 1997. MTHFR 677C→T mutation, folate intake, neural-tube defect, and risk of cardiovascular disease. *Lancet* 350(9078):603–604.

Winter RM, Knowles SAS, Bieber FR, Baraitser M. 1988. *The Malformed Fetus and Stillbirth. A Diagnostic Approach*. New York: John Wiley & Sons. P. 172.

Woolf CM, Turner JA. 1969. Incidence of congenital malformations among live births in Salt Lake City, Utah, 1951–1967. *Social Biology* 16(4):270–279.

World Atlas of Birth Defects. 2001. Available online at www.icbd.org/publicaiton.htm# WorldAtlasofBirthDefects.

World Health Organization (WHO). 1989. Glucose-6-phosphate dehydrogenase deficiency. *Bulletin of the World Health Organization* 67(6):601–611.

World Health Organization (WHO). 1996. *Control of Hereditary Diseases: Report of a WHO Scientific Working Group*. Geneva: WHO.

World Health Organization (WHO). 1997. Alwan AA, Modell B (eds.). *Community Control of Genetic and Congenital Disorders*. Alexandria, Egypt: WHO: EMRO Technical Publications Series.

World Health Organization (WHO). 1999. *Human Genetics: Services for the Prevention and Management of Genetic Disorders and Birth Defects in Developing Countries: Report of a Joint WHO/WOAPBD Meeting*. Geneva: WHO.

World Health Organization (WHO). 2000. Preventing congenital rubella syndrome. *Weekly Epidemiological Record* 75(36):290–295.

World Health Organization (WHO). 2001. *Assessment of Iodine Deficiency Disorders and Monitoring Their Elimination. A Guide for Program Managers*. 2nd edition. Pp. 1–122.

Wu Y, Zeng M, Xu C, Liang J, Wang Y, Miao L, Xiao K. 1995. Analyses of the prevalences for neural tube defects and cleft lip and palate in China from 1988 to 1991 [Article in Chinese]. *Hua Xi Yi Ke Da Xue Xue Bao* 26(2):215–219.

Wyss K, Guiral C, Ndikuyeze A, Malonga G, Tanner M. 1996. Prevalence of iodine deficiency disorders and goitre in Chad. *Tropical Medicine and International Health* 1(5):723–729.

Yamamuro T, Ishida K. 1984. Recent advances in the prevention, early diagnosis, and treatment of congenital dislocation of the hip in Japan. *Clinical Orthopaedics and Related Research* 184:34–40.

Yamashiro Y, Shimizu T, Oguchi S, Shioya T, Nagata S, Ohtsuka Y. 1997. The estimated incidence of cystic fibrosis in Japan. *Journal of Pediatric Gastroenterology and Nutrition* 24(5):544–547.

Yang H, Chung CS, Nemechek RW. 1987. A genetic analysis of clubfoot in Hawaii. *Genetic Epidemiology* 4(4):299–306.

Yusuf HK, Quazi S, Kahn MR, Mohiduzzaman M, Nahar B, Rahman MM, Islam MN, Khan MA, Shahidullah M, Hoque T, Baquer M, Pandav CS. 1996. Iodine deficiency disorders in Bangladesh. *Indian Journal of Pediatrics* 63(1):105–110.

Zhang SZ, Xie T, Tang YC, Zhang SL, Xu Y. 1991. The prevalence of chromosome diseases in the general population of Sichuan, China. *Clinical Genetics* 39(2):81–88.

Zlotogora J. 1997. Genetic disorders among Palestinian Arabs: 1. Effects of consanguinity. *American Journal of Medical Genetics* 68(4):472–475.

3

Interventions to Reduce the Impact of Birth Defects

The impact of birth defects in developing countries can be reduced through a series of interventions and eventually a comprehensive program that encompasses prevention, education about reproductive health, diagnosis, treatment, and rehabilitation. Several interventions presented in this chapter involve prevention of common birth defects and have been found to be affordable in even the poorest settings. These high priority interventions can be expanded as other health problems are resolved, as birth defects become a public health priority, and as additional resources become available. The health care provided to children and adults with birth defects should always be equitable with the care provided for other health conditions. In low-resource settings this may be very limited, but as the level of health care improves, the ability to diagnose and treat birth defects can be expanded and the quality of medical support for rehabilitation programs can be improved. Once health care has reduced infant mortality due to other causes, screening for genetic defects becomes cost-effective and can further reduce the impact of birth defects. Although the number and severity of birth defects pose a challenge to countries with limited health resources, the process of reducing the impact of birth defects can be undertaken in three stages:

1. Introduction of low-cost preventive interventions.
2. Provision of improved treatment for children and adults with birth defects.
3. Introduction of screening to identify genetic birth defects that can be prevented or treated.

Developing countries have a wide range of priorities, capacities, and resources for health care services. Successful implementation of each intervention requires that it be matched to the local setting. At each stage of development, health care services also need national leadership and coordination, surveillance to provide a sound evidence base for setting public health priorities, and monitoring of interventions to ensure their clinical- and cost-effectiveness.

BASIC REPRODUCTIVE CARE

Basic reproductive care, which includes family planning, and preconceptional, prenatal, and neonatal care, is the foundation for improving neonatal and infant mortality and reducing birth defects. As infant mortality rates fall, birth rates tend to decline because parents become increasingly confident that the children they conceive will survive childhood. This trend is strongest where family planning is accessible and effective.

Family Planning

The primary goal of family planning is to provide couples with the knowledge they need to make well-informed decisions concerning whether, when, and under what circumstances to have children. Accomplishing this goal involves education and assistance in preventing unintended pregnancies. Planning for a family of the desired size and preventing additional births can substantially reduce the number of children born with birth defects simply by reducing the total number of births. In addition, couples who have an established genetic risk of producing children with birth defects can choose whether to have any (or more) children (World Health Organization, 1997).

Preconceptional Care

Maternal education, literacy, and overall socioeconomic status are powerful influences on the health of both mother and neonate (Bicego and Boerma, 1993; World Bank, 1993; Rao et al., 1996; van Ginneken et al., 1996). Where both the formal education and the health education of girls are limited, there is an especially acute need for preconceptional health care, which aims to ensure that women and their partners achieve an "optimal state of physical and emotional health at the onset of pregnancy" (Wallace and Hurwitz, 1998).

Preconceptional care identifies risk factors for adverse birth outcomes, including birth defects, and provides the means to minimize those risks.

Identification of risk factors involves the following assessments (Moos, 1994):

- Medical history to identify preexisting medical conditions, such as insulin-dependent diabetes mellitus, epilepsy, and heart disease, that may pose a threat to the mother and the developing fetus; medications used by the mother; and exposure to rubella and other infectious diseases.
- Family history to identify birth defects in close family members.
- Reproductive history to identify risk factors that have contributed to previous poor pregnancy outcomes, some of which can be addressed through preconceptional and prenatal care.
- Nutritional profile to determine the overall nutritional status and intake of micronutrients, such as iodine and folic acid.
- Life-style profile to determine the potential for maternal exposure to infectious agents or recreational drugs such as alcohol.
- Maternal occupation should be evaluated for potential teratogenic exposures.

Preconceptional care advises on how to prevent certain birth defects that originate during the first weeks of pregnancy—often before a mother realizes she is pregnant. At 2 to 8 weeks' gestation, when embryonic cells are dividing rapidly and organ systems and body parts are beginning to differentiate, the embryo is particularly vulnerable to teratogens (Moos, 1994). For example, folic acid supplementation (discussed later in the chapter) is only effective in preventing neural tube defects (NTDs) when consumed during the periconceptional period.

Prenatal Care

An early prenatal visit permits the identification and review of risk factors for the pregnancy and prenatal diagnosis if the fetus is at high risk of having a birth defect. As noted above, this is too late for certain preventive measures such as increasing dietary consumption of folic acid to avoid NTDs.

Neonatal Care

Where possible, neonatal care should include a complete physical examination at birth (or prior to discharge for those born in a clinic or hospital) to diagnose detectable conditions. Early diagnosis followed by timely treatment can minimize some conditions and reduce disability. Infants with birth defects should receive the best care locally available. This will vary with local resources, the prevalence of specific birth defects, and the cost and effectiveness of potential interventions (Christianson et al.,

2000; World Health Organization, 1985, 1999b; Alwan and Modell, 1997). Low-cost rehabilitation may be less effective than prevention of birth defects, but it can reduce dependence and provide a better quality of life for affected individuals and their families.

> Recommendation 1. Basic reproductive health care services—an essential component of primary health care in all countries—should be used to reduce the impact of birth defects by providing:

- Effective family planning,
- Education for couples on avoidable risks for birth defects,
- Effective preconceptional and prenatal care and educational campaigns to stress the importance of such care, and
- Neonatal care that permits the early detection and best care locally available for management of birth defects.

LOW-COST PREVENTIVE STRATEGIES

These low-cost interventions to prevent birth defects have been found to be affordable in even the poorest settings. They address some important risk factors and involve family planning, public health campaigns, fortification of staple foods, maternal and child health, and infectious disease control.

Discouraging Pregnancy in Women Over 35

The simplest means of preventing Down syndrome and other chromosomal disorders such as trisomies 13 and 18 is to decrease the number of pregnancies among women older than 35 years. This is accomplished by making family planning widely available and providing information about what Down syndrome is and how it is caused (World Health Organization, 1997, 2000a). This strategy was shown to be effective in Europe between 1950 and 1975 when family planning programs were expanded and the birth prevalence of Down syndrome decreased from 2.5 to 1.0 per 1,000 live births (Modell and Kuliev, 1990).

> Recommendation 2. Women should be discouraged from reproducing after age 35 to minimize the risk of chromosomal birth defects such as Down syndrome.

Folic Acid Fortification

The predominant cause of NTDs is folate deficiency in the early weeks of pregnancy (Oakley, 1993). Randomized controlled trials in Europe showed that folic acid supplementation in early pregnancy reduced NTDs by 70 percent (MRC Vitamin Study Research Group, 1991) and 100 percent (Czeizel and Dudas, 1992). A randomized controlled trial from India was halted because of the ethical need to provide folic acid to all participants once its effectiveness had been established. The findings of that study supported the conclusion that folic acid deficiency is the predominant cause of NTDs (Indian Council of Medical Research, 2000). In a large, non-randomized community intervention study in a high-prevalence area (4 to 5 NTDs per 1,000 births) of China, pregnant women received daily supplements of 400 micrograms of synthetic folic acid before and during the first 28 days of pregnancy. This prevented 85 percent of NTDs among pregnant women taking folic acid more than 80 percent of the time (Berry et al., 1999) (see Box 3-1).

Although folic acid is present in leafy vegetables, legumes, and citrus fruits, it is unlikely that dietary advice alone can adequately increase con-

---

BOX 3-1 Preventing Neural Tube Defects with Folic Acid Supplementation in China

From 1993 to 1996, a large population-based observational study tested the ability of periconceptional folic acid supplementation to prevent neural tube defects (NTDs) in infants. The study was undertaken in two populations: one in northern China, where NTDs have a high prevalence (6.5 per 1,000 live births), and one in a southern region, where their birth prevalence is low (about 1 per 1,000). As described by Berry et al. (1999), 247,831 pregnant women were registered in the study (88 percent of pregnant women in the northern region and 90 percent of pregnant women in the southern region) in the 39 month study beginning in October 1, 1993. The users took 400 micrograms of folic acid daily on at least 80 percent of days of the periconceptional period; others were classified as nonusers, late users, or those who discontinued early. Infants with NTDs were identified by a population-based surveillance system in which photographs were taken of newborn infants of at least 20 weeks gestation and birth defects diagnosed by 6 weeks and of all stillborn infants.

In both regions, a higher rate of NTDs occurred among the infants and fetuses of women whose diets were not supplemented with folic acid, and the rate of NTDs decreased with increased use of folic acid. For northern women who took no folic acid, the rate of NTDs among fetuses or infants was 6.5 per 1,000 pregnancies, compared with 0.8 percent among southern women who took no folate. The rates of NTDs in the fetuses and infants of women receiving any additional folic acid were 1.3 (north) and 0.7 (south) per 1,000 pregnancies. The greatest reduction in NTDs occurred in women who took folic acid for more than 80 percent of the periconceptional period. Their fetuses and infants had similar low rates of NTDs (0.7 in the north, 0.6 in the south). The difference in background rates of NTDs in the two regions was concluded to be due in part to differences in dietary folic acid intake (Berry et al., 1999).

sumption of these foods by those at risk. The above studies led the United States to fortify cereal grains with synthetic folic acid to increase consumption of the nutrient by an average of 100 micrograms a day (Food and Drug Administration, 1996). Although this amount represents just one-quarter of the daily consumption recommended, it raised blood folate to levels that decreased NTDs by about 20 percent (Green, 2002; Oakley 2002a). The United Kingdom and Chile fortify at about twice the U.S. level. Since Chileans consume twice as much wheat as each of the other populations, the average woman in Chile is estimated to receive the recommended level of 400 micrograms of synthetic folic acid daily (Oakley, 2002a). Folic acid fortification is being introduced in several South and Central American countries, many of which already fortify wheat flour with other B vitamins. Folic acid is so inexpensive that the cost of the vitamin premixture hardly changes with its addition. In countries where folic acid fortification is not already under way, its cost is estimated at 0.1 percent of the total cost of flour.

Fortification overcomes the logistical problems of supplementation in early pregnancy as well as taking a complete regimen. However, almost universal coverage for women of reproductive age is relatively inexpensive. Fortification is recommended at a level of 240 micrograms per 100 grams of a widely consumed staple food (Oakley, 2002b). Supplementation is useful where fortification is not possible or is below the recommended level (Committee on Medical Aspects of Food and Nutrition Policy, 2000).

> **Recommendation 3. All women of reproductive age should routinely receive 400 micrograms of synthetic folic acid per day for the reduction of neural tube defects. This is best accomplished through fortification of widely consumed staple foods. Where fortification is not feasible or is incomplete, daily supplementation programs should be provided for women before and during pregnancy.**

Universal Salt Iodization

The primary cause of iodine deficiency disorders (IDDs) is insufficient iodine in the diet. The adult requirement for iodine can be met with 100 to 150 micrograms daily, and an additional 50 micrograms daily during pregnancy (Stanbury, 1998; World Health Organization, 2001). Correction of maternal iodine deficiency before conception is necessary to avoid adverse effects on the fetus. Measurement of urinary iodine is a convenient and reliable method for assessing iodine nutritional status in a community. This method is more accepted and considerably less expensive than the use of thyroid-stimulating hormone or other thyroid hormone measurements (Dunn et al., 1994; World Health Organization, 2001).

Iodine deficiency may be exacerbated by goitrogens, which interfere with the incorporation of iodine into thyroxine (Geelhoed, 1999). The effects of goitrogens can be mitigated by ensuring a more-than-adequate intake of iodine; avoiding consumption of thiocyanate-containing vegetable products such as cassava; and cooking potentially goitrogenic foods to reduce the goitrogen content (Bourdoux et al., 1982). Soaking foods is also effective in reducing the goitrogen level, but vitamin A and other nutrients are also lost in this process. Vitamin A deficiency can be addressed with dietary supplements (Vanderpas et al., 1993).

Iodine, a volatile trace element, is more abundant in the sea than on land. Except in certain geological regions (Li et al., 1989), iodine has been largely depleted from world soils (McClendon, 1939). Plants do not require iodine for healthy growth, and the amount of iodine in plants and animals generally reflects the low levels in soil. Thus to prevent iodine deficiency, most populations need supplementation (Hetzel and Maberly, 1986).

The accepted strategy for eliminating iodine deficiency is universal salt iodization (Stanbury, 1998), which is among the most cost-effective health interventions (World Bank, 1993). However, since this estimate does not encompass an assessment of the full impact of IDDs, the actual cost is likely to be lower (World Health Organization, United Nations Children's Fund, International Council for the Control of Iodine Deficiency Disorders, 1999). The customary level of fortification is 25–50 milligrams of iodine per kilogram of salt (World Health Organization, 1996b). The fortified salt product costs only slightly more ($0.02–$0.06 per person annually) than the unfortified product.

In populations with endemic cretinism and IDDs, iodized oil has been administered to entire populations as an emergency prophylactic and therapeutic (Delange, 1996; Geelhoed, 1999). In a Central African population in remote Congo, for example, an intramuscular injection of iodized oil was found to control goiter and cretinism and protect iodine stores for a period of 1 to 5 years, which reduces concerns about compliance (Geelhoed, 1999). Iodization of drinking water and bread has also been shown to provide a safe and cost-effective alternative in some settings (Elnager et al., 1997).

National leaders at the 1990 World Summit for Children set the goal of virtually eliminating this deficiency by the year 2000. In 1990, less than 20 percent of household salt was iodized, and more than one-third of the world's population was recognized as having inadequate dietary iodine. By 2002, more than 70 percent of household salt worldwide was iodized. Annually, this supplementation protects about 85 million infants, but another 35 million infants remain unprotected (Ramalingaswami, 2000). Figure 3-1 shows the percentage of house-

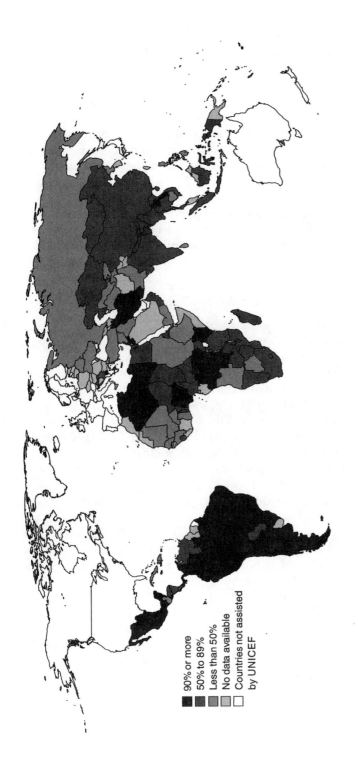

FIGURE 3-1 Distribution of households by their use of iodized salt.
SOURCE: United Nations Children's Fund, 2000a.

holds worldwide that use iodized salt, and efforts are under way to reach those households by 2005.

The rapid progress of the last decade has demonstrated the effectiveness of national "ownership" of the challenge (Ramalingaswami, 2000) and close collaboration among public, private, civic, and scientific groups to support the production of good-quality iodized salt, the delivery of *only* iodized salt, persistent market outreach to all parts of the country, periodic advocacy to sustain political commitment, and continued education to sustain public demand.

Recommendation 4. A program of universal fortification of salt with 25–50 milligrams of iodine per kilogram of salt used for human and animal consumption should be adopted to prevent iodine deficiency disorders.

Immunization Against Rubella

Rubella infections are common worldwide and are strongly teratogenic. Vaccination programs in several, mostly developed, countries prevent virtually all cases of congenital rubella. Some countries have immunized all young children, some have immunized prepubescent females, and some have used a combined approach—with measles-mumps-rubella (MMR) vaccine (Immunization Working Group, 2000; Massad et al., 1995). By 1996, 78 countries worldwide reported national rubella vaccination programs. Included among these were 43 percent of Latin American, 12 percent of Eastern Mediterranean, 5 percent of South East Asian, and 11 percent of the Western Pacific populations. Notably absent were African countries (Robertson et al., 1997).

The decision to introduce rubella vaccination into a country or region should be based on the susceptibility of women of childbearing age, the burden of disease due to congenital rubella syndrome (CRS), the strength of the measles immunization program, the infrastructure and resources for immunization, the record of injection safety, and other priority uses for limited health resources (World Health Organization, 2000b). In countries where more than 80 percent of the population is immunized for other childhood diseases, rubella should be included in the immunization program. In countries where immunization coverage is lower than 80 percent, overall coverage should be increased before introducing rubella immunization because vaccination can interrupt natural transmission during childhood and actually increase the number of women who are not immune (Banatvala, 1998). A vaccination strategy developed and implemented in Brazil was able to eliminate CRS in 2 years (see Box 3-2).

BOX 3-2 Rubella Vaccination in São Paulo, Brazil

Using a model based on epidemiological and cost-effectiveness data, public health officials in São Paulo, Brazil, developed and implemented a strategy for rubella vaccination in 1992. Children of 1 to 10 years of age were targeted for a mass vaccination, then all children were routinely immunized at 15 months of age. Researchers estimated that 96 percent of the target population in the State of São Paulo received MMR vaccine during the campaign.

Immediately after the campaign and again a year later, a rubella seroprevalence survey was conducted on a representative subset of about 3,000 children covered by the mass vaccination program. Blood samples from these children, randomly selected from 300 schools, were analyzed by enzyme-linked immunosorbent assay (ELISA) to estimate the age-dependent distribution of seroprevalence of antibody specific to the rubella virus. The average seroprevalence of rubella had increased from 0.40 to 0.97, while the number of confirmed cases of CRS had dropped from 16 in 1992, to 1 in 1993, to 0 in 1994.

SOURCE: De Azvedo Neto et al., 1994; Massad et al., 1994.

The most rapid reduction in CRS has been achieved with mass campaigns for all women of childbearing age. Checking for rubella antibodies before conception allows those who test negative to be immunized and those who test positive to be reassured. The benefits are considerable, while the main risk is the inappropriate reassurance of women who have false-positive tests (Tookey et al., 1991). All evidence indicates that rubella virus vaccine does not pose a risk to the fetus, so prior screening for pregnancy is unnecessary (Josefson, 2001; World Health Organization, 2000b). Vaccination of women of childbearing age against rubella has been shown to have a benefit-to-cost ratio of 11 to 1 in the United States (Hatziandreu et al., 1994) and a benefit-to-cost ratio of more than 1 in several developing-country studies (Hinman et al., 2002).

Eradication of rubella is feasible because it infects only humans and the vaccine is highly immunogenic, highly protective, affordable in all but the poorest countries, and can be administered in conjunction with measles and rubella vaccines and as part of a standard immunization schedule at 9 months of age (Plotkin et al., 1999). Eradicating rubella has not, however, been recognized as a priority in low-income countries (Banatvala, 1998). Combining rubella and measles vaccines can significantly reduce the cost of rubella immunization (Cutts and Vynnycky, 1999). In Latin America and the Caribbean, for example, 20,000 or more infants are born with CRS each year, yet a one-time mass immunization of all females aged 5 to 39 years could control both rubella and CRS (Hinman et al., 1998).

Surveillance of rubella and CRS following an eradication campaigns can be a challenge as rubella is often unreported and sometimes asymptomatic. Rubella epidemics are monitored using immunoglobulin M (IgM) testing in serum and saliva samples (Perry et al., 1993). Simple hearing tests for infants would improve case ascertainment (Plotkin et al, 1999), while testing all infants with microcephaly, developmental delay, hearing loss, microphthalmia, congenital cataracts, and congenital heart disease would capture a more complete estimate of CRS incidence.

> **Recommendation 5. Women should be vaccinated against rubella before they reach reproductive age to prevent congenital rubella syndrome.**

Preventing Other Congenital Infections

Primary prevention of maternal infection with herpes simplex virus and *Toxoplasma gondii* is the only way to prevent mother-to-child transmission of these agents.

Herpes simplex virus (HSV)

Where possible and safe, pregnant women with active genital herpes lesions at the time of delivery should deliver by cesarean section to decrease the risk of neonatal HSV. The risk is decreased to less than 10 percent if performed prior to the rupture of membranes (Nahmias and Schwahn, 1985).

Toxoplasmosis

Pregnant women can avoid exposure to *Toxoplasma gondii* by washing their hands after handling raw meat, cooking meat until well done, and avoiding contact with cat feces and soil, insects, or other material contaminated with cat feces (Essawy et al., 1990).

Limiting Alcohol Consumption

Alcohol consumption during pregnancy causes fetal alcohol syndrome, which is the most common preventable cause of mental retardation (Viljoen, 1999). A safe level of maternal alcohol use has not been established. The teratogenic risk of maternal binge drinking during pregnancy is uncertain, but studies suggest that a single heavy binge at a critical period of embryonic development can damage the fetus (Gladstone et al., 1996). Since the earliest weeks of pregnancy are critical for central nervous system development, all women should be strongly advised to avoid (Institute of Medicine, 1996) or minimize alcohol consumption before conception as well as during pregnancy. Where alcohol is recognized as an important public health problem, educational campaigns directed at schoolchildren, participants in family planning classes, and the general public should aim to increase public awareness of the risks of alcohol during pregnancy.

Recommendation 6. Education programs and public health messages should counsel women to limit or avoid alcohol consumption during pregnancy including during the early weeks.

Avoiding Teratogenic Medications During Pregnancy

Prevention of birth defects due to teratogenic medications such as anticonvulsants, anticoagulants, thalidomide, accutane, and misoprostol requires awareness of the consequences of their use on the part of medical workers and women of childbearing age. Educational campaigns, health messages, and preconceptional counseling on the prevention of birth defects should include information on medications to be avoided during periconception and pregnancy. In some cases, as with heparin versus other anticoagulants (Hardman et al., 1996), alternative medications can be substituted. Anticonvulsant monotherapy for epilepsy has been found to be associated with a lower rate of malformations than polytherapy (Adab et al., 2001, Kaneko et al., 1998).

Recommendation 7. Education programs and public health messages should educate health care providers and women of childbearing age about the importance of avoiding locally available teratogenic medications during pregnancy.

As with teratogenic medications, public awareness of the risks for birth defects associated with environmental pollutants is an important means of prevention. However, individuals may be powerless to avoid chemical pollutants that permeate their home or workplace. Exposure to such teratogens should be prevented through regulation of their manufacture, use, and disposal. Such reforms will require collaboration among the branches of government and, in some cases, international commitment.

Recommendation 8. Ministries of public health, in collaboration with other government departments in developing countries, should establish regulations to reduce occupational exposure to teratogens—such as mercury and other pollutants—and create programs to raise public awareness of the health risks, including birth defects, associated with these substances.

Summing Up

The burden imposed by birth defects justifies widespread implementation of the highly cost-effective interventions recommended above. Successful implementation of these interventions will require resources for personnel, training programs, and supplies of nutrients, vaccines, and medications.

> **Recommendation 9. Where possible, cost-effective interventions to prevent birth defects should be provided through public health campaigns and the primary health care system. The resources necessary for their success, including staff, training, and adequate supplies of nutrients, medicines, and vaccines should be provided as well.**

PROVISION OF IMPROVED CARE

The health care provided to children and adults with birth defects should always be comparable with the care provided for other medical conditions and the best possible for the resources available. In many settings this may be very basic, but even where health care resources are limited, affordable and effective options exist for the treatment and rehabilitation of those with birth defects. Early diagnosis—prenatal or neonatal—provides the best chance for effective treatment. Counseling of parents should also address future pregnancies and how the risk for a future pregnancy to involve a birth defect can be lowered.

Treatment

An important aspect of reducing the impact of birth defects is access to treatment. Although some disorders cannot be treated cost-effectively or at all, others can be corrected partially or entirely by therapies that are clinically- and cost-effective. Treatments can be made available by screening for patients with treatable conditions, then referring them to secondary and tertiary centers. These opportunities are frequently overlooked by policy makers and health professionals in developing countries, and access to treatment in many countries is limited (Christianson, 2000; World Health Organization, 1999).

Prenatal or early neonatal diagnosis can be important for scheduling surgery or initiating therapy before conditions become more severe or irreversible. While few tertiary centers in low-income countries can undertake complex surgery such as cardiac procedures for children with congenital heart disease, simpler surgical procedures are generally available but with limited access. The setting of priorities for the development of surgical capacity should be based on the resources required, current health care capacity, the availability and sustainability of technical expertise, and cost-effectiveness in comparison with other health care services.

Each country must establish clear priorities for the provision of treatments based on the cost-effectiveness of specific therapies and surgeries as compared with other health care services. This process is complicated by the lack of evidence on the cost-effectiveness of many services, including neonatal surgery, even in developed countries (Stolk et al., 2000). Long-term follow-up to estimate the lasting success of surgery and other therapies is complicated by the difficulty of identifying an outcome that is comparable for different surgeries and treatments. Moreover, generic quality-of-life measurements used for adults have to be adjusted to reflect children's understanding and perception. The following discussion presents therapies that are employed successfully in many developing countries.

Talipes or clubfoot

Infants with talipes include those whose deformity can be resolved through manipulation and passive stretching, and those who require surgery (Porter, 1987). In either case, early intervention is critical to correcting the condition and obtaining a foot that is supple, painless, plantigrade, and of normal shape and function. Serial manipulation, a gentle and gradual method of elongating the contracted tissues, should begin within a day or two of birth (Sinha, 1987; Alexander et al., 1999). By 12 weeks of age, the soft tissues of the infant foot are far less pliable, so only surgery can correct the condition (Sinha, 1987). For this reason, talipes can be considered an orthopedic emergency (Scott and Evans, 1997).

The principles of surgical treatment for talipes have been recognized for nearly 150 years: surgery should be early; it should correct the deformity; and the correction should be maintained—at first with a cast and later with a splint or brace worn at night (Porter, 1987). The surgical techniques employed depend on the severity of the condition, the age of the patient, and the health care setting (Alexander et al., 1999; Porter, 1987; Jellis, 1988). Early surgery may be appropriate for a child whose family is unlikely or unable to comply with routines for manipulation of the foot; however, the risk of injury during complex procedures increases significantly for very small feet (Turco, 1974). When manipulation fails, bone surgery can make the foot plantigrade, but this generally compromises mobility (Porter, 1987).

Most of the treatment of talipes in Africa is provided by medical officers without specialized training. In East Africa, for example, only 10 percent of children with talipes are likely to reach a specialist because of poor communications, travel expenses, and parental reluctance to leave family and crops. Patients who do reach surgeons often face delays in treatment due to the inadequate health care resources (Jellis, 1988). Efforts to over-come these challenges have met with variable success. A weekly "clubfoot clinic" established in a teaching hospital in Lusaka, Zambia, corrected 287 feet, 133 of them surgically over a 4-year period, with only eight relapses (Parekh, 1985). In this study, 95 percent of the patients attended the clinic regularly during treatment, and most returned for checkups even after full correction. In contrast, a program offered by a nonspecialist medical officer at a 78-bed rural mission hospital in Tanzania was considered unsuccessful because of poor parental compliance (Scott and Evans, 1997). Despite improvement in all cases, none of the 26 children attended over a sufficient period of time to be cured or referred for surgery. Other authors have also described low-cost, locally appropriate technologies for treating talipes (Sengupta, 1987; Eyre-Brook, 1986; Hadidi, 1974). Box 3-3 describes simple surgical techniques developed in Calcutta to correct talipes.

Parental education on the etiology and treatment of talipes is key to overcoming major barriers to compliance: successful treatments are avail-able; surgery may be required; and after correction, periodic checkups should continue until the child's growth is complete. Families of infants undergoing manipulative treatment of the foot need to understand the importance of regular cast changing and manipulation, as well as how to care for the cast and perform neurovascular checks on the immobilized foot (Alexander et al.,

---

BOX 3-3   Managing Talipes in India

In the course of 20 years, beginning in 1964, 5,312 patients with talipes were treated with a success rate of 85 percent at Calcutta's Institute of Child Health and Postgraduate Education. The hospital, an advanced center for the management of pediatric disorders, serves patients from urban slums and rural areas. Management costs were contained through the use of simple, effective methods to correct the disorder—percutaneous elongation of the Achilles tendon, plantar fasciotomy, and corrective plasters—which shortened hospital stays and minimized the number of visits required. Additional savings were achieved by using inexpensive, locally made materials and low-cost equipment. The program also educated medical and para-medical workers in neonatal and child care on the need for ensuring early treatment of talipes; addressed fear and apathy in affected children; and involved parents and the community in treatment and rehabilitation.

In India, walking barefoot or in sandals and squatting are central to daily life. Thus, along with the appearance of the foot, treatment was directed toward enabling the child to walk without shoes and to squat. Of the children who received treatment before 4 months of age, 85 percent were able to achieve these treatment goals, as were more than half of the children treated later in infancy but before they began to walk. The remaining children were not able to maintain the treatment schedule.

SOURCE: Sengupta, 1987.

1999). They should be encouraged to promote normal growth and development, including sitting up and crawling, while the foot is immobilized (Kryzer, 1991; Alexander et al., 1999). Postcorrection follow-up for talipes could be incorporated into local community-based rehabilitation or maternal and child health programs (Scott and Evans, 1997).

Cleft lip and/or cleft palate

Early establishment of feeding is a priority for neonates with cleft lip and/or cleft palate. Prenatal detection of the condition, available in some urban areas, can help parents to prepare for feeding and other special care of their child (Bender, 2000). Surgical repair of the lip can be done at 3 months and palatal repair at 6 months of age. This surgery, which is simple and effective, is available in several developing-country settings through the services of visiting surgeons supported by international foundations such as Operation Smile (see Box 3-4) and Medical Group Mission Christian Medical and Dental Society (Smith et al., 1991).

As children with cleft lip and/or cleft palate grow, their condition can cause a variety of physical, functional, and social problems. These can be minimized when treatment is available and when families, teachers, and the

---

BOX 3-4 Surgical Correction of Cleft Lip and/or Palate

The impact of this birth defect can be significantly decreased by a simple plastic surgery procedure that costs approximately $750, takes as little as 45 minutes, and can be performed in hospitals and clinics in developing countries. Operation Smile, a private, not-for-profit volunteer medical services organization, was founded in 1982 by a plastic surgeon and his wife, a nurse and clinical social worker. Operation Smile is based in Virginia. The organization offers facial reconstructive surgery mainly through periodic missions to more than 30 locations in 20 developing countries. For more complicated surgeries, sponsorships are arranged to bring children and young adults to the United States for treatment. In 1999, Operation Smile provided surgery and care for more than 5000 children in 18 countries and the United States.

The organization also provides education and training for physicians and other health care professionals in developing countries, with 2-year fellowships intended to develop local capacity for correcting craniofacial deformities. The annual Operation Smile Physicians' Training Program brings surgeons from around the world to the United States for training in specialized surgical skills. Since its inception in 1987, this program has been attended by more than 400 health care professionals. The *Cleft Lip and Cleft Palate Interdisciplinary Training Manual* and an accompanying CD-ROM series, produced by the organization in 1999, address the team approach to cleft lip and palate repair and are designed for use by both international volunteers and in-country health care professionals.

SOURCE: Operation Smile, 2001.

community are informed about the cause and difficulties associated with the condition. Support and education are key components of ongoing care (Chapados, 2000). Comprehensive treatment, which is not accessible for most developing country populations, can include speech and language therapy, preventive and restorative dental care, orthodontics, secondary surgery, otolaryngology for hearing problems, and psychological counseling (Cockell and Lees, 2000).

Isolated cases of cleft lip and palate show strong familial aggregation with a significant genetic component (Christenson and Mitchell, 1996). The risk of recurrence is, however, generally low. Surgical repair is generally effective (Czeizel and Hirschberg, 1997) and the isolated defect is not an indication for pregnancy termination (Czeizel and Hirschberg, 1997), but orofacial defects may be associated with congenital malformations of the limbs, spine, and cardiovascular system (Pilu et al., 1986). Fetal karyotyping can detect associated chromosomal anomalies or syndromes (Bender, 2000; Cockell and Lees, 2001).

Congenital heart disease (CHD)

In developed countries, CHD is diagnosed by ultrasound and repaired during infancy, but most developing countries lack the infrastructure necessary to treat this condition. Researchers estimate that hundreds of thousands of children are born each year with surgically treatable CHD. Most are not treated and die as children or teenagers (Cartmill et al., 1966; Rygg et al. 1971; Kirklin and Barrat-Boyes, 1993). However, hundreds of these children have been assisted without charge in developed countries or by traveling surgical teams supported by charitable organizations. One such organization, the Save a Child's Heart Foundation, has also assisted some institutions in developing countries in the establishment of CHD treatment capabilities (see Box 3-5) (Cohen et al., 2001).

Developmental dysplasia of the hip (DDH)

Early diagnosis of DDH and simple, noninvasive postural treatments can prevent a severe and crippling condition. Without these early treatments, true dislocation of the hip requires a series of complicated surgeries and rehabilitations, the results of which are frequently unsatisfactory. The most widely used diagnostic screen for DDH, the manual Ortolani-Barlow (O-B) test, is often included in a routine neonatal clinical examination in developed countries (Leck, 2000). Its usefulness depends on the skill and experience of the pediatrician, physical therapist, or orthopedic surgeon in identifying unstable hips, particularly those most likely to degenerate into full dislocation (Medbø, 1961; Leck, 2000). Ultrasound provides a similar

---

BOX 3-5   Treatment of Congenital Heart Disease

Many developing-country children die of simple congenital heart lesions that can be repaired with a high success rate and at relatively low cost. To expand the availability of cardiac care to such children, the Israel-based Save a Child's Heart Foundation established a program in 1996 to link Wolfson Medical Center, a state-run tertiary hospital in Holon, Israel, with partner institutions in low-income countries. Within 4 years, the program had established seven partner sites in six countries: Ethiopia, Nigeria, Tanzania, Moldova, the Palestine Authority, and China (in the provinces Hebei and Gansu). The Israeli hospital serves as a regional center, which provides care and training and promotes improved conditions at its partner sites.

At Wolfson Medical Center, 72 staff members—including pediatric specialists in cardiac surgery, cardiology, intensive care medicine, and anesthesiology—and 35 volunteers donate their time and services to treat patients. Use of the facilities is arranged, at reduced cost, through the government of Israel. During the first 4 years of the program, 360 children from partner sites received surgical treatment for CHD at Wolfson, and 26 surgeries were performed by volunteers at partner sites. In addition, with support from Israeli foreign-aid programs, 5 physicians and 10 nurses from various partner sites received training at Wolfson on caring for children with CHD.

The developing-country partner sites were chosen for equal partnerships with the project hospital to support the diagnosis, treatment, and follow-up of CHD cases. The qualifying partner institutions each had a cardiologist or pediatrician with an interest in cardiology, access to an echocardiology machine, the ability to establish a clinic that focuses on children with CHD and provides postoperative follow-up, and the laboratory capability to test for HIV and hepatitis and to monitor Coumadin levels. Partner sites are responsible for providing round-trip transport of surgical patients to Wolfson and follow-up care, including medications. Patient families contribute expertise demonstrates a way of providing surgical interventions for those who cannot afford them.

SOURCE: Cohen et al., 2001

---

detection rate but may have a higher false-positive rate in primary DDH screening.

Clinical examinations in industrialized countries have been shown to detect approximately three-quarters of neonates whose hips are or will become dislocated. If the identified neonates are treated promptly by splinting, about two-thirds will not develop DDH (Leck, 2000). This estimate is, however, complicated by high levels of false-negative and false-positive results. Fewer false positives are likely if the O-B test is conducted at 6 weeks of age because many hips that appear dysplastic at birth stabilize without treatment by that time. Treatment appears to be equally effective at 6 weeks and can be undertaken successfully in children up to 2 years old (Kim et al., 1990), often through noninvasive methods (Ramsey et al., 1976; Mendes and Roffman, 1980; Kim et al., 1990). Early treatment maintains the thighs in a flexed and partly abducted position so that the head of each femur remains deep within the acetabulum, encouraging it to encompass the femoral head more completely. To maintain this position, the thighs are splinted for weeks to months (up to a year). Two widely used methods are the Pavlik harness, which holds the legs in soft stirrups, and the von Rosen splint, a solid support. These splinting methods have not been compared through randomized trials, nor have they been developed for optimal performance (Leck, 2000). Either splint can cause ischemic or avascular necrosis of the femoral head, which is often accompanied by reduced femoral growth. This effect can be minimized by maintaining the hips in moderate, rather than extreme, abduction (Leck, 2000). Dislocated hips that fail to respond to early splinting and those detected and treated in older children can be managed with a range of surgical procedures, depending on the child's age and the degree of dislocation (Kim et al., 1990).

Oculocutaneous albinism

For affected children, the symptoms of the disorder can be treated, and health education can improve the home care (and, eventually, self-care) of affected children and dispel misconceptions that surround the condition.

Affected children are extremely sensitive to the sun and have poor vision. Sun protection is critical since those affected can be severely sunburned from minute-long exposures, which over time make them vulnerable to skin cancer. Covering the skin with long-sleeved shirts, long pants, and wide-brimmed hats helps protect from exposure to ultraviolet A (UVA) radiation. Sunscreens with a sun protection factor (SPF) rating of greater than 25 should be used at all times (King et al., 1996). Vision problems, such as hyperopia, myopia, and astigmatism, require correction to obtain the best possible visual acuity (King et al., 1996). Nearly every respondent among 138 school children with albinism in rural Zimbabwe reported problems in school due to poor vision (Lund, 2001). Yet most of these children can function in a regular classroom, provided the teacher and school attend to their special vision needs (King et al., 1996).

Adults with albinism frequently encounter social problems associated with their appearance, including difficulty in finding employment (Lund, 1998). A survey of attitudes toward people with albinism conducted in urban Soweto, South Africa, found that although they may be accepted in their community, people with albinism were regarded as abnormal and perhaps not fully human (Kromberg, 1992). Negative attitudes persist and are based on myths and superstitions concerning albinism, the most pervasive being that people with the condition do not die normally, but "vanish." Treatment of the condition and education of the public about the medical cause should be used to dispel this and other myths, and allow affected individuals to be accepted (and to accept themselves).

Recommendation 10. Children and adults with birth defects should receive the best medical care that is available in their setting, including, where possible, medication and surgery. Treatment should be undertaken as early as possible and be provided through an organized referral process.

Rehabilitation

Many infants with severe birth defects experience lifelong disability requiring long-term treatment or rehabilitation (Carey, 1992; World Health Organization, 1996a, 1999b). There are promising models of rehabilitation services for children with birth defects even in settings where professional resources are extremely limited. These models are based in communities: schools, hospitals and other institutions, and primary health care. The more comprehensive models are in the primary care system and are based on a national rehabilitation strategy. Although this report focuses on the care of infants and children with birth defects, it is important to recognize that rehabilitation programs are also needed for adults impaired by lifelong conditions. In many cases, appropriate education and rehabilitation for children and adults substantially increases their ability to function independently and contribute to family and community responsibilities.

Community-based rehabilitation (CBR)

CBR has been defined as a strategy in communities for the rehabilitation, equalization of opportunities, and social integration of people with disabilities (International Labor Organization, United Nations Educational, Scientific and Cultural Organization, and World Health Organization, 1994; United Nations Children's Fund and the Ministry of Education and Science, Spain, 1994). The strategy mobilizes local resources and enables people with disabilities and their communities to create their own solutions and programs for rehabilitation. It also addresses the isolation and stigmatization experienced by people with disabilities and encourages those with disabilities to live lives that are as normal as possible and are integrated into society. Disabled children are encouraged, where possible, to attend public schools with the goal of their not being limited by different social expectations or environmental constraints (Groce, 1999). The Jamaican program described in Box 3-6, is an example of how individuals with disabilities can be viewed as partners in national development.

Since 1983, WHO has produced training manuals for CBR workers and promoted CBR as the most appropriate model of rehabilitation for people with disabilities, including those due to birth defects (World Health Organization, 1980, 1993; Helander et al., 1989). While the WHO ap-

---

BOX 3-6 Community-Based Rehabilitation in Jamaica

Jamaica's first community-based rehabilitation program, 3D Projects ("Dedicated to the Development of the Disabled"), began in 1985. At that time, few services for people with disabilities existed outside the capital, Kingston. The program, established by a nongovernmental organization, gradually expanded, and now receives almost 25 percent of its budget from the government. In the late 1980s, two other CBR programs adopted the 3D model and extended services to other parts of the country. By the year 2000, all of Jamaica had CBR services available. The services available vary with the area, however, so that not all residents with disabilities are reached.

The 3D model involves several components, the majority of which are carried out by parents of children with disabilities and other community members. Identification and assessment of disabilities occurs mainly in the community health service in Kingston and in rural hospital clinics. There, a doctor or nurse practitioner works alongside community workers using basic assessments that have been standardized and validated in an international epidemiological study. A program plan is drawn up for each child, who is then assigned to a community worker in his area. The community worker designs a training program and, in some cases, basic physical therapy, and demonstrates the chosen activities to the mother or caregiver. The mother is expected to carry out the activities and exercises between weekly visits by the community worker. From time to time, the child's progress is reviewed in the clinic.

The 3D program also coordinates activities to strengthen family and community involvement in rehabilitation, including parent orientation sessions; community workshops; a prevocational adult-adolescent program; and the training of health care workers, police, social workers, and teachers.

The projected (though not achieved) budget for the four parishes of the 3D program for 1999 was approximately US$500,000. This funding supported the care of approximately 1000 children and adolescents at a cost of about US$500 per child annually.

SOURCES: Thorburn, 1993; Thorburn et al., 1992, 1993; Jonsson, 1994.

---

proach to CBR is largely home-based, model center-based approaches have also been developed (Werner, 1987).

The advantages of the CBR approach are its accessibility to low-income families and its ability to work with low-cost, locally available resources. The disadvantages are the lack of skilled resources, funds, and volunteered time; the difficulty of monitoring the quality of services and effectiveness in reaching the desired outcomes; and the inadequate opportunities for ongoing training and advancement of rehabilitation workers. Even with these drawbacks, CBR may be the most viable and cost-effective model for rehabilitative care in developing countries provided interventions are flexible, sensitive to cultural beliefs, appropriate to the country's current level of development, and compatible with local resources and development priorities.

School-based models

Educational opportunities for children with disabilities are limited in low-income countries. When available, they range from highly segregated, specialized residential and day schools to special classes in regular schools to a fully mainstreamed or inclusive education. Little information is available on the extent to which mainstreaming is practiced in low-income countries. Promotion of this approach began internationally following such agreements as the United Nations Educational, Scientific and Cultural Organization (UNESCO) Declaration of Education for All, which stipulates that all countries have a responsibility to provide equal access to education for children with disabilities as an integral part of the education system (Haddad, 1990; UNESCO and Ministry of Education and Science, Spain 1994). CBR and inclusive education appear to be mutually reinforcing, since CBR programs attempt to place children in regular schools, and teachers derive support from CBR workers when they accept children with disabilities (Thorburn, 2000). Box 3-7 describes school-based programs and other activities of the Bangladesh Protibondhi Foundation.

Reports from some low-income countries indicate that many schools do not have the facilities, trained teachers, or positive attitudes required to accommodate children with disabilities (Mariga and Phachaka, 1993). Given the already overcrowded environment of government schools in most low-income countries, a major commitment of resources is required to accommodate these children.

Institution- and hospital-based models

Institutional care and hospital-based services for children with birth defects are present in many low-income countries but serve only a small fraction of the children who need them. Rehabilitation specialists generally agree that institutional care should be discouraged because it promotes psychological dependence and prevents children from interacting with their peers and integrating into society. Perhaps the strongest disadvantage, however, is the cost. The monthly cost per child in an institution for disabled children in Harare, for example, was US$80 in 1990, a cost that exceeded the monthly income of the majority of Zimbabwean families (House et al., 1990).

Some institutions have supported community-based approaches, as described in Box 3-8. Institutions that previously offered long-term residential care have been converted to boarding schools for severely disabled children, who return to their families during school vacations. Institutions can also provide short-term rehabilitation for rural children who require surgery or the fitting of appliances. Hospital rehabilitation departments that traditionally focused on the short-term rehabilitation of patients with an acute

---

BOX 3-7   Rehabilitation Activities at Bangladesh Protibondhi Foundation

The Bangladesh Protibondhi Foundation (BPF), established in 1985, provides services and undertakes research for disabled children in Bangladesh. Key activities and achievements include:

Kalyani Special School in Dhaka was established for children with intellectual and motor disabilities. Children are first assessed at a clinic; then, infants can be enrolled in a mother-child early intervention program; children with cerebral palsy, speech and language problems, and behavioral problems such as autism can take classes; adolescent boys and girls are taught carpentry, weaving, and painting; and disabled and other children are educated at an affiliated school.

Dhamrai Rural School. Normal and intellectually disabled children attend this primary school 50 kilometers north of Dhaka. There are services for children with motor disabilities and sensory impairments, a mother-child early intervention program, and adult literacy programs for parents of disabled children.

Distance Training Packages. Pictorial manuals are developed to remind mothers who cannot come to a center regularly of the training they have received in handling or teaching their disabled child in motor development, speech and communication, cognitive development, and daily activities. An evaluation found these packages to be as effective as regular attendance at a center (McConkey and O'Toole, 1999).

Community-Based Rehabilitation. In collaboration with governmental and nongovernmental organizations BPF uses 10 questions and door-to-door screening to identify persons with disabilities and provides a professional assessment of those identified as disabled (Zaman et al., 1990).

Institute of Special Education is a postgraduate institute, approved in 1998 by the National University, which offers a one-year course that leads to a B.Ed. in special education.

Department of Special Education, Dhaka University, was founded in 1996 by BPF to train teachers of children with intellectual, visual, or hearing disabilities.

Research Program in Developmental Disabilities undertakes methodological research on screening and early assessment (Zaman et al., 1996); studies of the prevalence of and risk factors for developmental disabilities (Durkin et al., 2000); evaluation of distance training packages (McConachie et al., 2000); and development of training packages for teachers in schools that include disabled children with others (Munir and Beardslee, 1999).

---

disability, particularly those at the district and provincial levels, now provide technical, administrative, and training support to community-based programs through outreach activities. Rehabilitation villages have been constructed in rural hospitals so that disabled children and their caregivers can be accommodated for group activities and workshops.

Primary health care model

The most comprehensive CBR model is based in the primary health care system and is supported by a national strategy for rehabilitation of children and adults with disabilities including those from birth defects. Rehabilitation in Zimbabwe is an example of this model of care (see Box 3-8).

BOX 3-8 Rehabilitation of Disabled Children in Zimbabwe

Zimbabwe has a national strategy for rehabilitation of disabled children, which is coordinated through the health care system. Rehabilitation services are provided in communities, district hospitals, provincial hospitals, tertiary hospitals, and Harare Central Hospital. Tertiary and provincial-level hospitals are staffed by therapists and rehabilitation technicians, while district-level hospitals are staffed by rehabilitation technicians (who have 2 years of generic training in rehabilitation) with supervision by therapists at the provincial level. Community programs are staffed by village health workers with support from the district hospital staff (House et al., 1990). CBR has been introduced to the majority of the 55 districts in Zimbabwe, and urban programs have been established in the cities of Harare and Bulawayo. It is anticipated that every district will be covered by 2005 (Chidyausiku et al., 1998).

The cornerstone of Zimbabwean rehabilitative care is the Children's Rehabilitation Unit (CRU) at Harare Central Hospital. The CRU was established in 1986 to coordinate multidisciplinary treatment for children with disabilities and their families; provide tertiary-level assessment, diagnosis, and treatment planning for rehabilitation programs at provincial and district hospitals and in municipal clinics; disability and rehabilitation training for medical students, therapists, rehabilitation technicians, and nurses; maintenance of a computerized client register and database; and workshops to educate parents about specific disorders. These activities have increased awareness among health professionals of the problems facing children with disabilities and their families and of initiatives that might address them.

The main objective of the CRU is to support the development of CBR. Therefore, after initial assessment and training of a patient at the unit, ongoing therapy is carried out in the community. This accomplishes two goals: easier access for patients to rehabilitation services and facilitation of community-based support groups that can initiate self-help programs and lobby for disabled children at local government levels. The mothers have established a number of projects, based mainly on handicrafts, that provide them with regular income. Several groups have built day care centers and preschool facilities. The CRU provides weekly or fortnightly rehabilitation services.

The CRU staff organized the Zimbabwe Parents of Handicapped Children's Association, which has more than 4,500 members and branches throughout the country. The association advocates for children with disabilities and their families and addresses issues such as receiving priority in allocation of housing, obtaining access to special education for their children, developing income-generating projects, and addressing negative family and cultural attitudes toward people with disabilities.

SOURCES: Mariga and Phachaka, 1993; Zimbabwe Ministry of Education, Sports and Culture, 1998; Powell, 2000.

Psychosocial support

Birth defects have serious lifelong consequences for both the patient and the family. Those afflicted require psychological, emotional, and social support on a continuing basis; this support should include referral to and assistance from social services such as education and social welfare. Many birth defects lead to death in infancy or early childhood, so care of the patient may also include terminal or palliative care.

Depending on the setting, care may be provided by a nurse, physician, or other health worker trained to provide appropriate support (see Box 3-6) (Christianson et al., 2000). These caregivers must provide the best locally available care for the patient and the family (World Health Organization, 1999; Christianson et al., 2000), including addressing their concerns and uncertainties. Patient and parent support groups can provide mutual assistance and support (World Health Organization, 1999).

Recommendation 11. Parents of children with birth defects should be guided to organizations that provide rehabilitation for the child and psychosocial support for the child and family. Education policies at the national and local levels should ensure that all children, including those with birth defects, receive appropriate schooling.

SCREENING FOR GENETIC DISORDERS

Over the past four decades, infant mortality in developing countries has declined, though there is still room for considerable improvement (Table 3-1).

Once countries have successfully used the basic strategies of reproductive health care to reduce infant mortality, up to two-thirds of which is neonatal mortality (Hill, 1999), the more intractable causes of mortality and severe morbidity become the next challenge. Important among these are the more common genetic disorders for which screening becomes essential to further decrease infant mortality (World Health Organization, 2000a). Such programs are more demanding of resources and highly trained staff than are programs for basic reproductive health care; but, when introduced after basic reproductive health care services have reduced mortality, they too can be cost-effective. Screening programs were introduced in Cuba when the infant mortality rate (IMR), had been lowered to 19 per 1,000 live births (Heredero, 1992) and in Costa Rica (Saborio, 1992) at a similar IMR.

Genetic screening of populations identifies clinically normal individuals who have genotypes associated with a birth defect or who are at high risk of producing offspring with a birth defect. It aims to identify as many affected

TABLE 3-1 Improving Infant Mortality Rates in Developing Countries (1960–1999)

Country	Total Population, 1999 (thousands)	Infant Mortality Rate per 1,000 Live Births 1960	1999
Afghanistan	21,923	215	165
Albania	3,113	112	29
Algeria	30,774	152	36
Angola	12,479	208	172
Argentina	36,577	60	19
Armenia	3,525	38	25
Azerbaijan	7,697	55	35
Bangladesh	126,947	149	58
Barbados	269	74	14
Belarus	10,274	37	23
Benin	5,937	176	99
Bolivia	8,142	152	64
Bosnia and Herzegovina	3,839	105	15
Brazil	167,988	115	34
Bulgaria	8,279	49	14
Burkina Faso	11,616	181	106
Burundi	6,565	151	106
Cambodia	10,945	—	86
Cameroon	14,693	151	95
Central African Republic	3,550	187	113
Chad	7,458	195	118
Chile	15,019	107	11
China	1,266,838	150	33
Colombia	41,564	82	26
Congo	2,864	143	81
Congo, Democratic Republic	50,335	175	128
Costa Rica	3,933	80	13
Côte d'Ivoire	14,526	195	102
Croatia	4,477	70	8
Cuba	11,160	39	6
Czech Republic	10,262	22	5
Dominican Republic	8,364	102	43
Ecuador	12,411	107	27
Egypt	67,266	189	41
El Salvador	6,154	130	35
Eritrea	3,719	170	66
Ethiopia	61,095	180	118
Gabon	1,197	171	85
Georgia	5,006	52	19
Ghana	19,678	127	63
Guatemala	11,090	136	45
Guinea	7,360	215	115
Haiti	8,087	169	83

(continued)

TABLE 3-1 continued

Country	Total Population, 1999 (thousands)	Infant Mortality Rate per 1,000 Live Births 1960	1999
Honduras	6,316	137	33
Hungary	10,076	51	9
India	998,056	146	70
Indonesia	209,255	128	38
Iran	66,796	164	37
Iraq	22,450	117	104
Jamaica	2,560	58	10
Jordan	6,482	97	29
Kazakhstan	16,269	55	35
Kenya	29,549	122	76
Korea, Democratic People's Republic	23,702	85	23
Korea, Republic of	46,480	90	5
Kyrgyzstan	4,669	135	55
Lao People's Democratic Republic	5,297	155	93
Latvia	2,389	35	17
Lebanon	3,236	65	28
Lesotho	2,108	137	93
Liberia	2,930	190	157
Libya	5,471	159	19
Lithuania	3,682	52	18
Madagascar	15,497	219	95
Malawi	10,640	205	132
Malaysia	21,830	73	8
Mali	10,960	293	143
Mauritania	2,598	180	120
Mexico	97,365	94	27
Moldova, Republic of	4,380	64	27
Mongolia	2,621	—	61
Morocco	27,867	132	45
Mozambique	19,286	180	127
Myanmar	45,059	169	79
Nepal	23,385	212	75
Nicaragua	4,938	130	38
Niger	10,400	211	162
Nigeria	108,945	123	112
Pakistan	152,331	139	84
Panama	2,812	58	21
Papua New Guinea	4,702	137	79
Paraguay	5,358	66	27
Peru	25,230	142	42
Philippines	74,454	80	31
Poland	38,740	62	9
Romania	22,402	69	21
Russian Federation	147,196	48	18
Rwanda	7,235	124	110

TABLE 3-1   continued

Country	Total Population, 1999 (thousands)	Infant Mortality Rate per 1,000 Live Births 1960	1999
Saudi Arabia	20,899	170	20
Senegal	9,240	173	68
Sierra Leone	4,717	220	182
Slovakia	5,382	33	9
Somalia	9,672	175	125
South Africa	39,900	89	54
Sri Lanka	18,639	83	17
Sudan	28,883	123	67
Syria	15,725	136	25
Tajikistan	6,104	95	54
Tanzania	32,793	142	90
TFYR (The Former Yugoslav Republic of) Macedonia	2,011	120	22
Thailand	60,856	103	26
Togo	4,512	158	80
Tunisia	9,460	170	24
Turkey	65,546	163	40
Turkmenistan	4,384	100	52
Uganda	21,143	133	83
Ukraine	50,658	41	17
Uruguay	3,313	48	15
Uzbekistan	23,942	84	45
Venezuela	23,706	56	20
Vietnam	78,705	147	31
Yemen	17,488	220	86
Yugoslavia	10,637	87	20
Zambia	8,976	126	112
Zimbabwe	8,976	97	60

SOURCE: United Nations Children's Fund, 2000b.

individuals as possible, but screening alone does not detect all individuals at high risk. Diagnosis usually follows a positive screening test and it provides a high level of accuracy. Examples of screening programs include those for α-thalassemia in Asian populations, β-thalassemia in Mediterranean populations, sickle cell disorder (SCD) in African populations, glucose-6-phosphate hydrogenase (G6PD) deficiency in female relatives of a patient with the deficiency, and chromosomal abnormalities in women over 35 years of age.

Genetic screening programs can involve preconceptional detection of risk factors associated with birth defects, also prenatal and neonatal screening and diagnosis of birth defects. The criteria for establishing screening programs for genetic disorders are presented in the next section, followed by a discussion of the important role of genetic counseling in any screening effort. The specific goals and methods of preconceptional, prenatal, and neonatal screening for birth defects follow, then ethical considerations of screening, diagnosis, and prevention or treatment.

Criteria for Establishing Genetic Screening Programs for Genetic Disorders

Screening programs need to be tailored to the health priorities of each community as determined by epidemiology, demographics, resources, and the capacity of health care services. The following prerequisites guide the determination of which birth defects can benefit from genetic screening (Simpson and Golbus, 1992; Cuckle and Wald, 2000):

- **The target condition is serious and relatively common.** Since individuals with less serious birth defects can live fulfilling lives, the conditions that are appropriate for screening are those that are serious or life threatening.
- **Screening takes place at the best possible time.** While screening may be conducted in the preconceptional, prenatal, or neonatal periods, the earlier a diagnosis is made, the more opportunities may be available to prevent a birth defect or minimize its severity.
- **The screening assay clearly distinguishes between individuals who have the condition and those who do not.** Since each birth defect is relatively rare, the assay should have a low false-positive rate.
- **Effective and acceptable management strategies are available.** Population screening and prenatal diagnosis for α- and β-thalassemia, sickle cell anemia, and phenylketonuria (PKU) are appropriate because there are management strategies for each.
- **The program is cost-effective.** Although the technology is available to screen for many disorders, not all screening is likely to be cost-effective in a given population or health care setting.

Thalassemia

β-Thalassemia major is easy to diagnose, and effective—though costly—treatment is available. Blood transfusions combined with iron chelating therapy allow many people with the disorder to survive into their twenties and thirties. A more expensive and higher-risk option—stem cell transplant from bone marrow or cord blood—can cure the disorder but is not affordable in low-income populations. Without diagnosis and treatment, patients with β-thalassemia major usually die early in childhood; thus, the population prevalence of β-thalassemia is a fraction of the birth prevalence, and the cost of treating the few people who survive to adulthood is low. Where diagnosis and treatment for β-thalassemia are available, patients survive longer, the population prevalence increases, and national treatment costs rise. Screening and control programs have significantly reduced the birth prevalence of β-thalassemia in Greece (Loukopoulous, 1996), Iran (see Box 3-9), and Sardinia (Cao et al., 1991, 1996).

A premarital screening program in the Aegean region of Turkey tested nearly 10,000 couples over 4 years and found a β-thalassemia trait prevalence of 2.6 percent in that population. Prenatal screening of the same population identifies at-risk couples who are offered prenatal diagnosis

---

BOX 3-9   Control of Thalassemia in Iran

Iran has a population of 67 million, is a middle-income country, and spends 6 percent of its gross national product on health services, which are exemplary (United Nations Children's Fund, 2000; Shadpour, 1994). Thirty years ago, there were no services for the diagnosis and treatment of severe birth defects such as thalassemia. The carrier frequency of β-thalassemia varied from 1 to 12 percent in different Iranian population subgroups. The birth prevalence was 0.74 per 1,000, which resulted in 1,250 new cases each year, a number that was increased by the high level of parental consanguinity. Affected infants did not survive so the population prevalence was a fraction of the birth prevalence, and the national cost of care was negligible. As diagnosis and treatment of birth defects with blood transfusions and iron chelating therapy became available, however, 90 percent of patients survived into their late teens, the population prevalence increased, and the national cost of care for thalassemia treatments rose. Bone marrow transplants, which can cure β-thalassemia, are not affordable or available in Iran (World Health Organization, 2000a). With 15,000 registered thalassemia patients, the national cost of thalassemia care reached approximately US$200 million per year, 0.28 percent of the national health budget. Without a national program for prevention, the cost was estimated to increase to US$700 million, or 1 percent of the current national health budget (World Health Organization, 2000a).

When the national program for prevention was introduced, it halved the number of annual births of children with thalassemia. Beginning in endemic areas, then nationally, mandatory screening and counseling became required of couples before marriage. Where both partners have thalassemia minor, they are advised against marriage. Prenatal diagnosis by private health services became available in 1994 for private patients with plans to extend it to the National Health Service (Angastiniotis et al., 1995; World Health Organization, 2000a). Because of the heavy burden of thalassemia on affected individuals, their families, and society, policy makers introduced a decree that provided access for all to prenatal diagnosis and the option for termination of pregnancy in the first 120 days for severe birth defects, which include thalassemia.

SOURCE: Modell, Royal Free and University College London Medical School, personal communication.

and, in the case of pregnancies with β-thalassemia major, pregnancy termination (Keskin et al., 2000). Hospital-based prenatal screening programs in Thailand (Jaovisidha et al., 2000) identify pregnancies at risk for α- and β-thalassemias. At-risk couples are offered prenatal diagnosis and, if severe thalassemia is diagnosed, the option to terminate the pregnancy.

Sickle cell disorder

More than 60 percent of all births of children with SCD or other major hemoglobin disorders occur in Africa, the region with the most limited resources for addressing these conditions (Angastiniotis et al., 1995). Thus, while there are treatments for SCD, cost-effective measures to educate at-risk couples and communities about SCD and reduce the number of children born with sickle cell anemia (HbSS) appear to be important, but have not been recognized as a priority. To date, Cuba is the only country in Latin America (Angastiniotis et al., 1995) that has initiated a comprehensive control program for SCD; it is described in Box 3-10.

As with thalassemia, primary prevention of SCD can be achieved through preconceptional genetic screening and counseling of couples at risk for having a child with the disease, while secondary prevention can be provided through prenatal screening and counseling, which may be followed by prenatal diagnosis and the possibility of terminating affected pregnancies. Where genetic screening is not available, couples who have given birth to a child with SCD should be advised on the risk for future pregnancies.

Where screening for sickle cell trait and disease is undertaken, neonatal screening permits the early treatment of SCD. It also provides the opportunity to educate parents on the care of affected children and the risk for future pregnancies. The potential harm that could result from false-positive and false-negative results should be carefully considered.

Treatments for SCD include measures to reduce the symptoms and severity of anemia and prevent potentially fatal infections (penicillan prophylaxis and pneumococcal vaccine), to which SCD patients are especially susceptible (Lees et al., 2000; Steensma et al., 2001). Hydroxyurea can prevent vaso-occlusive crises (Koren et al., 1999), but the drug is expensive (Charache et al., 1995; Kate, 2001; Davies and Oluhohungbe, 2002). Bone marrow transplantation is available in high-resource settings (Kate, 2001), but rarely in developing countries. Some homozygotes with high levels of fetal hemoglobin may need little more than long-term folate supplementation, while others require aggressive supportive care, frequent hospitalizations, pain relief, and transfusions (Steensma et al., 2001). Pulmonary symptoms require immediate attention since acute chest syndrome is a major cause of death (Vichinsky et al., 1997).

BOX 3-10   National Genetic Screening in Cuba

In 1981, in response to the increasing proportion of infant mortality and morbidity attributable to birth defects and the local development of appropriate diagnostic screening tests, Cuba initiated a national program for the prevention of locally prevalent disorders (Heredero, 1992). The program was designed to screen for SCD in all pregnant women; detect major fetal anomalies, including NTDs, with maternal α-fetoprotein screening and fetal ultrasonography; provide cytogenetic diagnosis for women of advanced maternal age (over 40 years of age); screen newborns for phenylketonuria (PKU); and provide genetic counseling services at the primary care level (Granda et al., 1991; Heredero, 1992).

Initial coverage of the population was limited, but by 1990, services were available countrywide. The program operates in hospital-based genetic centers in all 14 provinces, seven regional cytogenetic laboratories, and specialized laboratories in designated academic and tertiary care centers. The National Centre of Medical Genetics was established in Havana for research and the training of specialists in genetic health care (Heredero, 1992).

Since 1988, more than 90 percent of all pregnancies have been screened for risk of SCD (Heredero, 1992). Annually about 300 at-risk couples are identified, counseled, and offered prenatal diagnosis. In 1989, it was estimated that the program had reduced the number of infants born with SCD by 30 percent (Granda et al., 1991). In Havana the birth prevalence of NTDs has been reduced by almost 90 percent since 1982 (Rodriguez, et al., 1997). Approximately 500 fetuses with anomalies are detected annually with ultrasonography. Between 1984 and 1990, chromosomal abnormalities were detected in 202 fetuses; the parents were offered counseling, and in 90 percent of the cases, they requested termination of the pregnancy (Heredero, 1992). Newborn screening for PKU covered 85 percent of births by 1990, and screening for congenital hypothyroidism was introduced in 1992 (Granda et al., 1991; Heredero, 1992; Rodriguez et al., 1997).

Cuba provides an example of how a low-income country has been able to target priority health conditions and establish an effective program to screen for key genetic disorders.

In some developing countries, SCD goes largely undiagnosed and leads to high mortality during the first 5 years of life (Akinyanju, 1989; Angastiniotis et al., 1995). Under such circumstances, health education is a priority, since there is no chance for prevention or treatment in populations where SCD is not recognized and diagnosed. Where treatment for SCD is unavailable—such as in tribal areas of Maharashtra, India—a combination of health education and genetic screening has been suggested as the most effective means of reducing the impact of SCD (Kate, 2001).

Glucose-6-phosphate dehydrogenase deficiency

The primary effects of G6PD deficiency are hematological (Verjee, 1993), so most interventions focus on reducing the occurrence and severity of hemolytic crises. These episodes can be precipitated by infections such as hepatitis or pneumonia; exposure to certain chemicals and oxidative medications, including some antimalarial drugs; and consumption of fava beans (Chatterjea, 1966; Meloni et al., 1992; Beutler, 1994; Verjee, 1993). Avoiding these triggers for hemolysis requires that affected persons be diagnosed and counseled. Occasionally those with the Mediterranean form of the deficiency and those in hemolytic crisis require a blood transfusion.

Elevated bilirubin levels, elevated reticulocyte count, and low red blood cell count and hemoglobin levels are signs of G6PD deficiency. In the neonate, hyperbilirubinemia may be severe and, if left untreated, can cause bilirubin encephalopathy. Screening tests—fluorescent spot test, ascorbate cyanide test, MTT staining test, methemoglobin reduction methods, and dye decolorization (Verjee, 1993)—are quick, easy, inexpensive, and suitable for large populations. The diagnosis is confirmed by enzyme assay (Meloni, 1992), but the definitive assay requires laboratory equipment that is not usually available in the countries where G6PD deficiency is common.

Cystic fibrosis

Screening the family members of a patient with cystic fibrosis (CF) can detect the CF gene in 60–90 percent of carriers (Grody et al., 2001), which allows informed reproductive choices to be made (Frossard et al., 1999). An early diagnosis is key for prevention of CF since many high-risk couples have a second affected child before the diagnosis has been established for the first child (Rabbi-Bortolini et al., 1998). Prenatal screening programs have not become routine even in developed countries (Haddow et al., 1999).

The most important diagnostic test for CF in developing countries is the sweat electrolytes test (Mahashur, 1993). Screening tests include DNA testing, fecal fat, upper gastrointestinal and small bowel series, and measurement of pancreatic function. In Latin America, CF is underdiagnosed because of high mortality rates from pulmonary and gastrointestinal diseases and limited access to the sweat test (Macri et al., 1991).

Ideally, treatment of CF would involve a multidisciplinary team (physician, physiotherapist, nutritionist, and social worker) to provide conventional therapy (antibiotics, pancreatic enzyme replacement by ingestion of capsules with meals, and nutritional support) and treatment for CF-associated complications (Mahashur, 1993; Zar et al., 1998). Such an intensive approach is not available or cost-effective in many settings.

Phenylketonuria

Screening for PKU is done with the relatively inexpensive Guthrie test on filter paper blood specimens. The timing of the screening is critical, so the specimen should be obtained in the hospital of birth as close to discharge as possible. Because second tests are unlikely to detect new cases, resources are best directed at improving the primary screening (Cunningham, 2000). In countries where the incidence of PKU is relatively high, such as Estonia (Ounap et al., 1998), and Latvia (Lugovska et al., 1999)—1 per 6,010 and 1 per 8,700 respectively—there are mass screening programs, while in countries, such as South Africa, where the incidence is low (Hitzeroth, 1995)—1 per 20,000—there are more pressing health priorities. The number of infants born at home and thus not diagnosed is undetermined.

The mainstay of treatment is a phenylalanine-restricted diet. By limiting daily consumption to only 250–500 milligrams of phenylalanine per day, a positive nitrogen balance and safe plasma levels of phenylalanine can be maintained. The amino acid supplements, which are taken with vitamin and mineral supplements are not palatable, which makes compliance with the restricted diet difficult (Cunningham, 2000; Poustie and Rutherford, 2001). The diet should begin as soon after birth as possible and be continued as long as the patient is able to comply. While a phenylalanine-restricted diet has been shown in nonrandomized studies to reduce blood phenylalanine levels and improve IQ and neuropsychological outcome, the evidence is inadequate for determining a safe upper level of phenylalanine and when, if ever, dietary restrictions can be relaxed (Poustie and Rutherford, 2001).

Because early dietary treatment has proven successful, affected women now become potential mothers (Cunningham, 2000). Avoiding mental retardation and other problems in their offspring requires that they resume the restricted diet prior to and throughout pregnancy to avoid phenylalanine levels that would be toxic to the fetus and cause severe mental retardation, birth defects, heart disease, and low birth weight.

Hemophilia A and B

Because hemophilias A and B are relatively uncommon, prenatal screening should be restricted to families with a history of the disorder. A fetal blood sample can be used for diagnosis of genetic disorders of red cells, white cells, or platelets and for identification of clotting factor deficiencies. Amniocentesis, chorionic villus sampling, or a placental biopsy are used to obtain cells for cytogenetic or biochemical analysis and to isolate fetal DNA (Weatherall and Letsky, 2000). Male patients with severe hemophilia are often diagnosed shortly after birth because of an extensive cephalohematoma or profuse bleeding at circumcision. Neonates suspected of having hemophilia should receive screening tests for hemostasis, including a platelet count, bleeding time, and blood clotting ability (Handin, 1998).

Treatment is complicated and expensive, which limits its usefulness for most developing countries. In Turkey, a program using intermediate concentrates rather than high-purity concentrates or recombinants and a twice-weekly regimen (instead of three times a week) reduced the cost of therapy (Kavakli et al., 1997). A rehabilitation center in India has reported a program for preventing and treating acute hemarthrosis in which the patient is taught a series of exercises that facilitate absorption of the hematoma to improve joint range and strengthen muscles, which reduces the frequency of bleeding (Kale, 1999).

Many centers have organized home care programs so that patients can administer their own factor VIII infusions with the onset of symptoms (Handin, 2001). Local health clinics can give injections to hemophiliacs. Home and local care spare limited health personnel resources and solve problems of transportation and absenteeism from school and work. Hemophiliacs are at high risk for HIV/AIDS and hepatitis B if a safe supply of blood products is not maintained. An alternative may be to import blood products.

Genetic Counseling

Counseling, an integral component of screening for genetic risk, assists couples or mothers by educating them about genetic risks and reproductive choices, thereby allowing them to make free and informed decisions (Hogge and Hogge, 1996; Biesecker, 2001). Prior to screening, counselors describe the conditions that can be identified and the available screening tests, diagnostic methods, and options for preventing or treating birth defects. The limitations of screening tests are explained, along with the goal of identifying high-risk pregnancies that may require invasive follow-up tests to obtain a diagnosis. Women or couples who do not see an advantage in having the diagnosis or do not wish to confront the options raised by the results of the screening process may decline to be screened. If they request screening, the counselor explains the test results and answers questions. When counseling those who had a positive screening test, the counselor provides information on the diagnosis, etiology, prognosis, and consequences; describes options for prevention; and responds to questions or concerns.

Counselors must be able to obtain accurate information and communicate clearly and respectfully. Printed explanations can be used as a reference and to convey information to family and friends. The counselor should avoid judgments and provide factual knowledge that empowers women or couples to make their own decisions. Counseling those with a previous abnormal pregnancy can be particularly challenging because anxiety can interfere with the ability to understand and retain information. These cases may require extra time to review the genetic history and answer questions. Where possible, families need to be reassured that they could not have prevented an abnormal pregnancy and to receive guidance on the risk for future pregnancies. When a birth defect does not carry a risk for future pregnancies, counseling can relieve much of the anxiety.

With appropriate training, a variety of health care professionals may serve as genetic counselors. In some settings, primary care workers are well positioned to counsel because they are known in the community, which can increase the trust and respect with which they are received (Christianson et al., 2000). Regardless of their previous medical qualifications, genetic counselors need to be trained and tested in the content and delivery of information. The content of each consultation should be documented and monitored. Genetic counselors provide an important linkage between health care and the social, religious, and legal underpinnings of society, which together determine the availability of reproductive choices.

Preconceptional Screening

Preconceptional screening has the advantage of identifying and counseling couples at high risk for producing a child with a birth defect before conception. The screening has three components: recording and evaluation of a genetic history, laboratory testing where indicated, and counseling. Genetic histories can identify clinically normal couples at risk for passing an inherited birth defect to their offspring and carriers of abnormal recessive genes who are at risk of passing a disorder to their children. Individuals at high risk can be screened and, if determined to be at risk, should receive counseling and other appropriate care (see Box 3-11).

A genetic history explores whether a couple is at risk for inherited disorders or for chromosomal abnormalities or mutations that could result in birth defects. Maternal age over 35 years is the most common risk factor for chromosomal abnormalities. Paternal age over 40 years increases the risk of certain dominant mutations (McIntosh et al., 1995). Exposure to mutagenic agents should also be determined. Abnormal reproductive outcomes (repeated spontaneous abortions, stillbirths, and infants born with birth defects) among first-degree relatives (siblings, parents, offspring), second-degree relatives (uncles, aunts, nephews, nieces, and grandparents), and third-degree relatives (first cousins) are reviewed. Identification of second- and third-degree relatives with birth defects generally does not increase a couple's risk significantly unless the couple is consanguineous. The ethnic origin of each potential parent should be noted because of the higher risk for certain birth defects among particular groups. Genetic histories can be recorded efficiently using a questionnaire that requires only positive responses (Simpson and Golbus, 1992).

Preconceptional screening of national populations or high-risk groups has been undertaken in countries where serious recessive birth defects are

---

BOX 3-11   Indications for Preconceptional Genetic Consultation

- Indication
  - Previous pregnancy history
  - Fetal demise
  - Recurrent pregnancy loss
- Previous child with a genetic disorder
  - Chromosomal: Down syndrome
  - Structural: NTD, dwarfism
  - Metabolic: neonatal or early childhood death, ambiguous genitalia
  - Hematologic: anemia, bleeding disorder
  - Mental retardation
- Family history of genetic disorder
  - Bleeding disorders: hemophilia
  - Neurological disease: muscular dystrophy, myotomicdystrophy
  - Mental retardation: fragile (X) syndrome
  - CF
- Risk associated with ethnic origin
  - African: Sickle cell anemia
  - Mediterranean: β-thalassemia
  - Oriental: α-thalassemia and β-thalassemia
  - Ashkenazi Jewish: Tay-Sachs disease
  - French-Canadian: Tay-Sachs disease
- Maternal medical disorders
  - Diabetes
  - PKU
- Maternal medications
  - Anticonvulsants
  - Anticoagulants
  - Lithium
  - Thalidomide
  - Accutane
  - Any chronically used medication
- Socially used drugs
  - Alcohol
  - Cocaine

SOURCE: Adapted from Hogge and Hogge, 1996.

---

prevalent, a reliable test is available, and the condition is amenable to prevention. Conditions that are common in the developing world and amenable to prevention include thalassemia and SCD. National screening is performed in Greece, Iran (see Box 3-9), Sardinia, and Cyprus for β-thalassemia and in Cuba for SCD (see Box 3-10). Family planning services provide an ideal setting for genetic screening and the use of genetic histories for the preconceptional prevention of birth defects.

Prenatal Screening and Diagnosis

Prenatal screening identifies pregnancies at high risk for genetic disorders but is not able to exclude the possibility of a birth defect. Prenatal diagnosis, which generally follows a positive result from prenatal screening, determines with more certainty the presence or absence of a birth defect. Prenatal screening programs can effectively address populations at high risk for Down syndrome, NTDs, and single-gene disorders (Baird, 1999). Screening and diagnosis take place before 20 weeks' gestation to allow parents to consider the option of pregnancy termination in the case of severe birth defects or to plan the time and place of delivery in cases where surgery is necessary at birth. The following procedures are widely used in developed countries for diagnosis and are increasingly available in the larger cities of developing countries.

Maternal serum screening

Identification of those at risk for Down syndrome, NTDs, and other fetal abnormalities should involve noninvasive screening methods for those at low risk—younger couples with no family history of these disorders. Elevated levels of α-fetoprotein in maternal serum are associated with NTDs and fetal anomalies. This single screen can identify more than 90 percent of first-occurring NTDs in a family, missing only 10–15 percent of all cases (Ross and Elias, 1997), which are closed NTDs. Because elevated α-fetoprotein levels also occur in cases of fetal death, underestimates of gestational age, or multiple gestations, an elevated result is often followed with a repeat test (before 18 weeks' gestation) and with ultrasonography. If these methods do not find a reason for the elevated α-fetoprotein level, amniocentesis can be used to obtain amniotic fluid for assays of α-fetoprotein and acetylcholinesterase. In the US about 3–5 percent of the latter procedures lead to diagnosis of an NTD.

Measuring levels of human chorionic gonadotropin, unconjugated estriol, α-fetoprotein, and sometimes inhibin A helps in the detection of Down Syndrome. The "quadruple screen" a noninvasive test (Ross and Elias, 1997; Wald et al., 2003), identifies women at elevated risk of carrying a fetus with Down syndrome. Only this selected group (rather than all) then undergoes the invasive procedures, amniocentesis or chorionic villus sampling, to obtain a definitive diagnosis.

Fetal ultrasonography

Ultrasound technology can be used to identify signs or markers indicating increased risk of a birth defect (e.g., screening for nuchal translucency and Down syndrome) or to detect structural malformations in the fetus (e.g., diagnosis of open NTDs). For most high-risk couples, the report of normal ultrasound findings provides considerable relief.

Screening for structural malformations is done at 18–20 weeks' gestation, when fetal abnormalities are large enough to be recognized. Although ultrasonography can detect more than 200 different fetal abnormalities, its appropriate use is limited to those conditions that can be addressed with an effective intervention. Depending on the setting, these conditions may include serious abnormalities that cause a severe disability for which termination of pregnancy is generally agreed to be justified, fatal abnormalities in which termination of pregnancy avoids waiting until the end of an unproductive pregnancy, and abnormalities where arrangements need to be made for treatment of the neonate immediately after birth. This option is offered only after appropriate, nondirective counseling.

Ultrasound technology is not universally available for population screening because of its expense and requirement for trained staff, but it is increasingly available in the larger cities of developing countries. The quality of screening varies widely with the experience of the operator and the resolution obtainable by the equipment. Ultrasound-based prenatal screening programs need to be carefully planned and monitored to ensure they are appropriate, viable, and cost-effective. The basic requirements for a cost-effective program include well-maintained instruments, staff who are fully trained in the instrumentation, guidelines on the number and timing of ultrasound examinations, a protocol or checklist of conditions to be examined, and guidelines on the level of screening for each condition. Screening services must also be adequately supported with counseling services and with diagnostic services for cytogenetic, biochemical, and molecular genetic analyses, all of which also have to be monitored for their cost and effectiveness. It is important to develop and refine pilot screening projects before implementing ultrasound screening nationwide. Well-planned screening programs are likely to be cost-effective since the treatment and rehabilitation of individuals with severe birth defects are expensive and since many couples choose to terminate a pregnancy if a severe birth defect is identified (Baird, 1999).

Amniocentesis and chorionic villus sampling

These sampling procedures provide cells of fetal origin that can used to identify a chromosomal condition by karyotyping or DNA analysis or a genetic disorder by enzymatic or DNA analysis. Amniocentesis involves the aspiration of amniotic fluid and is the most commonly used procedure. Chorionic villus sampling (CVS) involves aspiration of villi using a flexible cannula passed through the uterine cervix or a hollow needle inserted into the maternal abdomen. Both procedures are guided by ultrasound. Amniocentesis is usually undertaken in the fourteenth to sixteenth week of pregnancy, while CVS can be performed from the beginning of the tenth week until the end of the twelfth week of gestation.[1] Both amniocentesis and CVS have very high detection rates for chromosomal abnormalities—the principal goal of such sampling. Since second-trimester amniocentesis is easier to perform than CVS, particularly for inexperienced operators, it is the more widely used procedure. CVS can, however, be performed earlier in the pregnancy (Gosden et al., 2000).

Amniocentesis or CVS is typically offered for pregnancies at increased risk for chromosomal abnormalities—risks that once were determined solely by advanced maternal age and previous adverse obstetric history but are now increasingly identified by abnormal maternal serum markers and ultrasonographic evidence of early fetal abnormalities (Ross and Elias, 1997; Yang et al., 1999). Fetal karyotyping following amniocentesis is successful virtually 100 percent of the time, and the diagnosis is available in the sixteenth to nineteenth week of gestation. Because of the significant risk of maternal mortality and other major complications of abortion at this stage of pregnancy, early amniocentesis procedures have been developed with the aim of diagnosing severe birth defects prior to 15 weeks' gestation. Although these techniques make amniocentesis at 11 to 12 weeks' gestation possible, this approach is not generally recommended because it is associated with a higher failure rate, greater fetal loss, and increased birth prevalence of talipes compared with standard amniocentesis (Gosden et al., 2000).

For single-gene disorders such as the thalassemias, SCD, and CF, diagnostic testing of amniotic fluid or chorionic villi is appropriate where there is a family history of such disorders or as a follow-up for high-risk pregnancies identified in a screening test.

Neonatal Screening

Although neonatal screening generally plays a smaller role than prenatal screening, it provides an important opportunity to identify birth defects early in the neonatal period and be able to initiate therapy or surgery early in life. Early, appropriate treatment can prevent or reduce some lethal or disabling sequelae of birth defects. For neonates born in hospitals, screening should occur before they leave. Even when little can be done to help the infant, accurate diagnosis of birth defects can alert parents to the risks they may face in future pregnancies.

In Southeast Asian populations in which G6PD deficiency is common it can also be accompanied by neonatal jaundice and kernicterus. In these

---

[1]A 10-week gestation corresponds to 8 embryonic weeks after conception.

populations, early neonatal screening for G6PD deficiency is important. Affected infants are monitored for several weeks with regular tests of the bilirubin level (Weatherall and Letsky, 2000).

For PKU, congenital hypothyroidism, and other inherited metabolic defects, neonatal screening is the only screening available and it allows early dietary intervention for PKU and thyroid replacement therapy for hypothyroidism, both of which are critical to avoid mental retardation. Neonatal diagnosis of congenital hip dislocation provides the best chance for correcting this disorder through noninvasive techniques.

Ethical Considerations

Prevention, diagnosis, and treatment of birth defects can all benefit from the application of genetic knowledge when appropriate consideration is given to the following principles (World Health Organization, 1997):

- Respecting the autonomy of individuals and protecting those with diminished autonomy;
- Giving the highest priority to the care and welfare of individuals;
- Maximizing the benefits and minimizing the harm and cost to individuals; and
- Treating individuals with fairness and equity, and distributing the benefits and burdens of health care impartially.

Women and couples have the right to be appropriately informed and counseled about the screening services provided, to choose whether to accept them, and to receive continuing support independently of their choice. Before undergoing a screening test, they should be informed of the severity and frequency of occurrence of the birth defect being screened for, the detection rate for the test, the probability of being affected if the result is positive, the follow-up diagnostic test, and the choices available if the diagnostic test is also positive. If one choice is to terminate the pregnancy, this should be made clear, because some women or couples may not wish to face that choice. There is agreement in many countries that pregnancy termination must not be offered for the purpose of gender selection (Wald et al., 2000).

The entire population of a country or region should be offered the most effective and safe screening service possible, provided it is affordable and judged to be cost-effective compared with alternative screening methods. Priority should be given to genetic tests involving birth defects that impose the heaviest burdens on the population as a whole. In particular, efforts should be directed at the primary care level toward improving access to genetic screening where it has been judged to be cost-effective (World Health

Organization, 1997). Access to diagnostic procedures that are expensive or hazardous should be limited to those for whom the risk for the birth defect justifies the expense and the risk involved in the diagnosis (Wald et al., 2000). A genetic screening service should have the resources to provide all components of screening: testing, patient information, staff education, counseling, diagnostic and treatment services, monitoring, and quality and cost control (Wald and Hackshaw, 2000).

The results of genetic tests should be provided with supportive counseling that does not direct women or couples toward either continuing or terminating a pregnancy when the fetus is afflicted with a severe genetic disorder. Genetic data should be used only to benefit members of a family or ethnic group—it should never stigmatize or discriminate against them—and should be treated as confidential at all times (World Health Organization, 1997).

Summing Up

Genetic screening services provide an opportunity to profoundly reduce the impact of birth defects in developing countries. Such services are, however, expensive for countries with limited resources for health care because they require highly trained staff, sophisticated equipment, and the support of diagnostic and counseling services. Even after the initial high cost to establish such services, continued delivery of good quality services requires ongoing staff training and rigorous maintenance of the equipment. There is, however, a time for each country when more affordable interventions have substantially reduced infant and neonatal mortality due to more preventable conditions and birth defects become a priority. By that time treating birth defects can be taking up a substantial and increasing share of health costs and hospital beds, and genetic screening—for common and severe conditions—has been found, even by countries with limited resources, to be cost-effective relative to other health interventions.

Examples of national genetic screening programs that have been discussed in this chapter are found in Cyprus, Greece, Iran, and Sardinia for thalassemia, and in Costa Rica and Cuba for a wider set of locally prevalent genetic disorders. There are more examples of genetic screening programs that have been undertaken in regions of a country, such as the Northern Province of South Africa. Each country will have its own timing on the introduction of genetic screening programs, which is influenced by national and local priorities, the prevalence of preventable birth defects in the population, health care capacity, financial and human resources, and the ability to dedicate substantial additional resources. For many countries, this is likely to become important when other health interventions have reduced the infant mortality rate to the range of 20–40 per 1,000 live births.

Recommendation 12. Countries with comprehensive systems of basic reproductive health care that have lowered infant mortality rates to the range of 20 to 40 per 1,000 can further reduce infant mortality by establishing genetic screening programs. These programs should address severe, locally prevalent conditions with clear screening and diagnostic tests; effective, acceptable strategies for prevention or treatment; and be cost-effective. Counseling, with the goal of enabling individuals to make free and informed health care decisions, including the choice, where legal, to terminate a pregnancy in the case of a severe birth defect, should be integral to all screening and diagnostic programs.

NATIONAL COORDINATION, SURVEILLANCE, AND MONITORING

The impact of individual birth defects and of birth defects in the aggregate must be known with some accuracy if priority needs are to be identified and addressed. Epidemiological data can establish the prevalence and health burden associated with birth defects and provide information for establishing priorities for interventions. Regular surveillance provides trends and monitors the clinical- and cost-effectiveness of interventions. The assessment of neonatal mortality due to birth defects is difficult and expensive, however, since most deliveries in developing countries take place at home, and infant deaths that occur during or shortly after childbirth are rarely recorded in official statistics. As a result, data on total infant mortality and mortality due to birth defects vary widely and are almost certainly underestimates.

Developing countries differ widely in their needs and resources for the establishment of data systems. Further, establishment of a monitoring system competes for limited resources with interventions to reduce birth defects. However, even relatively simple efforts to monitor the birth prevalence of common birth defects (see Box 3-12), along with associated death and disability, can highlight priority areas and changes in those areas over time. This information is key to identifying priority interventions and to their success over time.

Recommendation 13. Collection of epidemiological data on birth defects is necessary to understand the extent of the problem and identify intervention priorities. Depending on the infant mortality rate, the capacity of the health care system, and the resources available, countries should incrementally develop the following:

• National demographic data on neonatal and infant mortality and morbidity,

---

**BOX 3-12   Community-Based Genetic Screening Services in
Rural South Africa**

In 1985 only 25 percent of the 5,000 patients seen at genetic clinics were black
South Africans, who at that time constituted 75 percent of the population. Limited
epidemiological information was available on this population. In 1989, surveillance
of birth defects was introduced in a rural hospital in Northern Province, one of the
poorest in South Africa. The birth prevalence of severe birth defects was higher than
that observed in industrialized countries. Three more common conditions included
NTDs (3.6 per 1,000 live births), Down syndrome (2 per 1,000 live births), and
oculocutaneous albinism (0.7 per 1,000 live births) (Jenkins, 1990; Christianson and
Kromberg, 1996).

In the early 1990s, genetic services were introduced through seven hospitals that
were visited regularly and others that were networked into the program. The sisters
(senior nurses) at the participating hospitals were trained to recognize patients with
a birth defect and refer them to outreach genetic clinics. Almost 1,800 patients were
evaluated: a birth defect was diagnosed in 66 percent of the patients, an undifferen-
tiated disability in 30 percent, and an acquired disability in 4.6 percent.

When the genetic clinics became oversubscribed in mid-1993, a primary care
facility for patients with common birth defects was established at each participating
hospital. This facility was integrated with secondary medical, paramedical, social,
and educational services and referred patients and specimens to tertiary-level services. It was staffed by the sisters who received additional training on patient care,
with the oversight of a hospital medical officer. Patients requiring specialist care
were seen at the hospital genetic clinics. Patients with Down syndrome, NTDs, and
oculocutaneous albinism comprised 25 percent of the birth defects caseload (Christianson et al., 2000).

Stillbirths and neonates with lethal birth defects were documented with full clinical notes, including photographs and chromosomal analysis. These notes were reviewed at subsequent genetic outreach clinics, and the parents were counseled.
Genetic counseling and ongoing psychosocial support were provided for patients
and their families by the sisters. Screening for birth defects was limited to the examination of newborns prior to discharge and the use of family histories to trace family
members at increased risk of being affected or being carriers. While limited in funding and capacity, this program provided significantly improved services for rural
patients with birth defects.

SOURCE: Christianson et al., 2000.

- Data on causes of death,
- Documentation of birth defects using standardized protocols for diagnosis, and
- Ongoing monitoring of the common birth defects in a country or region.

Many organizations and parts of government can contribute to the
strengthening of health care in developing countries. National leadership

and coordination of these organizations and capabilities can vastly improve the quality and equity of health care, including reproductive health care and care of birth defects.

Recommendation 14. Each country should develop a strategy to reduce the impact of birth defects, a framework of activities by which this can be accomplished, and the commitment of health leaders to accomplish these goals.

National programs of basic reproductive health should collect and interpret surveillance data, set uniform standards for the training and performance of health care providers, and foster communication among health care providers, researchers, and policy makers.

Recommendation 15. Each country should strengthen its public health capacity for recognizing and implementing interventions that have proven effective in reducing the impact of birth defects. This includes monitoring and tuning interventions for clinical- and cost-effectiveness in the local setting.

CONCLUSION

Despite the existence of low-cost interventions for preventing and treating a number of birth defects, the human, economic, and social burdens associated with these conditions remain high. Obstacles to improving care for birth defects include financial constraints; lack of knowledge on the part of health care workers; poor access to medical facilities; and issues surrounding ethnicity, language, religion, and culture. Governments must be educated on the cost-effectiveness of reducing the impact of birth defects through proven methods of prevention and care, which can be adapted to local resources and needs. Providing the best possible care for patients with birth defects begins with the recognition that such care may require significant financial commitment and that the care that can be provided will vary with the setting (World Health Organization, 1985, 1997, 1999; Carey, 1992).

Robust programs of basic reproductive health care and public health campaigns provide a framework for new efforts to reduce the impact of birth defects. Reducing the impact of birth defects in developing countries can be approached through a three-stage process. The first stage of the process involves low-cost interventions to prevent specific birth defects. The second stage addresses improved treatment and rehabilitation for those with birth defects. Although generally more costly than the first stage preventive interventions, reducing the disease burden for those with birth defects, is key to providing equitable health care as these individuals can suffer from both the burden of disease and an associated burden of lost social and economic opportunity. The third stage is important for countries with comprehensive systems of basic reproductive health care and lower IMRs. The screening and diagnosis of genetic disorders can further reduce infant mortality when they are tailored to national health priorities and address common and severe birth defects that can be accurately detected and effectively prevented or managed. Counseling, with the goal of enabling individuals to make free and informed health care decisions, is an essential part of screening and diagnostic programs.

REFERENCES

Adab N, Winterbottom J, Tudur C, Williamson PR. 2001. Common antiepileptic drugs in pregnancy in women with epilepsy. *Cochrane Database of Systematic Reviews* (2):1–14.

Akinyanju OO. 1989. A profile of sickle cell disease in Nigeria. *Annals of the New York Academy of Sciences* 565:126–136.

Alexander M, Ackman JD, Kuo KN. 1999. Congenital idiopathic clubfoot. *Orthopaedic Nursing* 18(4):47–55; quiz 56–58.

Alwan AA, Modell B. 1997. Community control of genetic and congenital disorders. Technical publication series, No 24. Alexandria, Egypt: World Health Organization Regional Office for the Eastern Mediterranean.

Angastiniotis M, Kyriakidou S, Hadjiminas M. 1988. The Cyprus Thalassemia Control Program. *Birth Defects Original Article Series* 23(5B):417–432.

Angastiniotis M, Modell B, Englezos P, Boulyjenkov V. 1995. Prevention and control of haemoglobinopathies. *Bulletin of the World Health Organization* 73(3):375–386.

Baird PA. 1999. Prenatal screening and the reduction of birth defects in populations. *Community Genetics* 2(1):9–17.

Balgir RS, Murmu B, Dash BP. 1999. Hereditary hemolytic disorders among the Ashram school children in Mayurbhanj district of Orissa. *Journal of the Association of Physicians of India* 47(10):987–990.

Banatvala JE. 1998. Rubella—could do better. *Lancet* 351(9106):849–850.

Bender PL. 2000. Genetics of cleft lip and palate. *Journal of Pediatric Nursing* 15(4):242–249.

Berry RJ, Li Z, Erickson JD, Li S, Moore CA, Wang H, Mulinare J, Zhao P, Wong LC, Gindler J, Hong S, Correa A. 1999. Prevention of neural-tube defects with folic acid in China. *New England Journal of Medicine* 341(20):1485–1490.

Beutler E. 1994. Glucose–6–phosphate dehydrogenase deficiency. *Blood* 84(11):3613–3636.

Bicego GT, Boerma JT. 1993. Maternal education and child survival: A comparative study of survey data from 17 countries. *Social Science and Medicine* 36(9):1207–1227.

Biesecker, BB. 2001. Goals of genetic counseling. *Clinical Genetics* 60(5):323–330.

Bourdoux P, Seghers P, Mafuta M, Vanderpas J, Vanderpas-Rivera M, Delange F, Ermans AM. 1982. Cassava products: HCN content and detoxification processes. In DeLange F, Iteae FB, Ermans EM (eds.). *Nutritional Factors Involved in the Goitrogenic Action of Cassava.* Ottawa: International Development Research Center. P. 51.

Cao A, Rosatelli C, Pirastu M, Galanello, R. 1991. Thalassemias in Sardinia: Molecular pathology, phenology, phenotype–genotype correlation, and prevention. *American Journal of Pediatrica Hematology/Oncology* 13(2):179–188.

Cao A, Rosatelli MC, Galanello R. 1996. Control of beta–thalassaemia by carrier screening, genetic counselling and prenatal diagnosis: The Sardinian experience. *Ciba Foundation study group* 197:137–151; discussion 151–155.

Carey JC. 1992. Health supervision and anticipatory guidance for children with genetic disorders (including specific recommendations for trisomy 21, trisomy 18, and neurofibromatosis I). *Pediatric Clinics in North America* 39(1):25–53.

Cartmill TB, DuShane JW, McGoon DC, Kirklin JW. 1966. Results of repair of ventricular septal defect. *Journal of Thoracic and Cardiovascular Surgery* 52(4):486–501.

Chapados C. 2000. Experience of teenagers born with cleft lip and/or palate and interventions of the health nurse. *Issues in Comprehensive Pediatric Nursing* 23(1):27–38.

Charache S, Terrin ML, Moore RD, Dover GJ, Barton FB, Eckert SV, McMahon RP, Bonds DR. 1995. Effect of hydroxyurea on the frequency of painful crises in sickle cell anemia. Investigators of the Multicenter Study of Hydroxyurea in Sickle Cell Anemia. *New England Journal of Medicine* 332(20):1317–1322.

Chatterjea JB. 1966. Haemoglobinopathies, glucose–6–phosphate dehydrogenase deficiency and allied problems in the Indian subcontinent. *Bulletin of the World Health Organization* 35(6):837–856.

Chidyausiku S, Munandi J, Marasha M, Mbazo D, Mhuri F, Oppelstrup H, Nleya C. 1998. *Community-based Rehabilitation Programme in Zimbabwe*. Sida Evaluation 98/15, Department for Democracy and Social Development. Stockholm, Sweden: Sida.

Christianson AL. 2000. Medical genetics in primary health care. *Indian Journal of Pediatrics* 67(11):831–835.

Christianson AL, Kromberg JR. 1996. Maternal non-recognition of Down syndrome in black South African infants. *Clinical Genetics* 49(3):141–144.

Christianson AL, Mitchell LE. 1996. Familial recurrence–pattern analysis of non-syndromic isolated cleft palate—a Danish registry study. *American Journal of Medical Genetics* 58(1):182–190.

Christianson AL, Venter PA, Modiba JH, Nelson MM. 2000. Development of a primary health care clinical genetic service in rural South Africa—the Northern Province Experience, 1990–1996. *Community Genetics* 3(2):77–84.

Cockell A, Lees M. 2000. Prenatal diagnosis and management of orofacial clefts. *Prenatal Diagnosis* 20(2):149–151.

Cohen AJ, Tamir A, Houri S, Abegaz B, Gilad E, Omohkidion S, Zabeeda D, Khazin V, Ciubotaru A, Schachner A. 2001. Save a child's heart: We can and we should. *The Annals of Thoracic Surgery* 71(2):462–468.

Committee on Medical Aspects of Food and Nutrition Policy. 2000. Folic acid and the prevention of disease. *Reports on Health and Social Subjects* 50:1–101.

Cuckle HS, Wald N. 2000. Principles of screening: Tests using single markers. In Wald N, Leck I (eds.). *Antenatal and Neonatal Screening*, 2nd edition. New York: Oxford University Press. Pp. 274, 473, 510.

Cunningham G. 2000. Phenylketonuria and other inherited metabolic defects. In Wald N, Leck I (eds.). *Antenatal and Neonatal Screening*, 2nd edition. New York: Oxford University Press. Pp. 353–369.

Cutts FT, Vynnycky E. 1999. Modelling the incidence of congenital rubella syndrome in developing countries. *International Journal of Epidemiology* 28(6):1176–1184.

Czeizel AE, Dudas I. 1992. Prevention of the first occurrence of neural–tube defects by periconceptional vitamin supplementation. *New England Journal of Medicine* 327(26): 1832–1835.

Czeizel AE, Hirschberg J. 1997. Orofacial clefts in Hungary. Epidemiological and genetic data, primary prevention. *Folia phoniatrica et logopaedica* 49(3–4):111–116.

Davies S, Oluhohungbe A. 2002. Hydroxyurea for sickle cell disease. *Cochrane Database of Systematic Reviews*, Issue 4.

De Azevedo Neto RS, Silveira AS, Nokes DJ, Yang HM, Passos SD, Cardoso MR, Massad E. 1994. Rubella seroepidemiology in a non-immunized population in São Paulo, Brazil. *Epidemiology and Infection* 113(1):161–173.

Delange F. 1996. Administration of iodized oil during pregnancy: A summary of the published evidence. *Bulletin of the World Health Organization* 74(1):101–108.

Dunn JT. 1994. Societal implications of iodine deficiency and the value of its prevention. In Stanbury JB (ed.). *The Damaged Brain of Iodine Deficiency.* New York: Cognizant Communications. Pp. 309–314.

Durkin MS, Khan NZ, Davidson LL, Huq S, Munir S, Rasul I, Zaman SS. 2000. Prenatal and postnatal risk factors for mental retardation among children in Bangladesh. *American Journal of Epidemiology* 152(11):1024–1033.

Elnager B, Eltom M, Karlsson FA, Bourdoux PP, Gebre–Mehdin M. 1997. Control of iodine deficiency using iodination of water in a goiter endemic area. *International Journal of Food Sciences and Nutrition* 48(2):119–127.

Essawy M, Khashaba A, Magda A, el–Kholy M, Elmeya S, Samy G. 1990. Study of congenital toxoplasmosis in Egyptian newborns. *Journal of the Egyptian Public Health Association* 65(5–6):669.

Eyre–Brook AL. 1986. An appropriate approach to orthopaedics in developing countries. *International Orthopedics* 10(1):5–10.

Frossard PM, Lestringant G, Girodon E, Goossens M, Dawson KP. 1999. Determination of the prevalence of cystic fibrosis in the United Arab Emirates by genetic carrier screening. *Clinical Genetics* 55(6):496.

Geelhoed GW. 1999. Metabolic maladaptation: Individual and social consequences of medical intervention in correcting endemic hypothyroidism. *Nutrition* 14(11–12):908–932.

Gladstone J, Nulman I, Koren G. 1996. Reproductive risks of binge drinking during pregnancy. *Reproductive Toxicology* 10(1):3–13.

Gosden C, Tabor A, Leck I, Grant A, Alfirevic Z, Wald N. 2000. Amniocentesis and chorionic villus sampling. In Wald N, Leck I (eds.). *Antenatal and Neonatal Screening,* 2nd edition. New York: Oxford University Press. Pp. 470–516.

Granda H, Gispert S, Dorticos A, Martin M, Cuadras Y, Calvo M, Martinez G, Zayas MA, Oliva JA, Heredero L. 1991. Cuban programme for prevention of sickle cell disease. *Lancet* 337(8734):152–153.

Green NS. 2002. Folic acid supplementation and prevention of birth defects. *Journal of Nutrition* 132(8 suppl):2356S–2360S.

Groce NE. 1999. Disability in cross-cultural perspective: Rethinking disability. *Lancet* 354(9180):756–757.

Grody WW, Cutting GR, Klinger KW, Richards CS, Watson MS, Desnick RJ. 2001. Laboratory standards and guidelines for population-based cystic fibrosis carrier screening. *Genetics in Medicine* 3(2):149–154.

Haddad E. 1990. *World Declaration Education for All.* Paris: United Nations Educational, Scientific and Cultural Organization.

Haddow JE, Bradley LA, Palomaki GE, Doherty RA, Berhardt BA, Brock DJ, Cheuvront B, Cunningham GC, Donnenfeld AE, Erickson JL, Erlich HA, Ferrie RM, FitzSimmons SC, Greene MF, Grody WW, Haddow PK, Harris H, Holmes LB, Howell, RR, Katz M, Klinger KW, Kloza EM, LeFevre ML, Little S, Loeben G, McGovern M, Pyeritz RE, Rowley PT, Saiki RK, Short MP, Tabone J, Wald NJ, Wilker NL, Witt DR. 1999. Issues in implementing prenatal screening for cystic fibrosis: Results of a working conference. *Genetics in Medicine* 1(4):129–135.

Hadidi H. 1974. Management of congenital talipes equinovarus. *Orthopedic Clinics of North America* 5(1):53–58.

Handin RI. 1998. Disorders of coagulation and thrombosis. In Fauci AS, Eugene B, Isselbacher KJ, Wilson JD, Martin JB, Kasper DL, Hauser SL, Longo DL (eds.). *Harrison's Principles of Internal Medicine*, 14th edition. Vol. 1. New York: McGraw–Hill. Pp. 737–738.

Hardman J, Goodman A, Gilman L, Limbird L. 1996. *Goodman and Gilman's: The Pharmacological Basis of Therapeutics*, 9th edition. New York: McGraw-Hill Professional.

Hatziandreu EJ, Brown RE, Halpern MT. 1994. *A Cost Benefit Analysis of the Measles–Mumps-Rubella (MMR) Vaccine: Final Report*. Arlington, VA: Battelle.

Helander E, Mendis P, Nelson G. 1989. *Training Disabled People in the Community*. Geneva: World Health Organization.

Heredero L. 1992. Comprehensive national genetic program in a developing country—Cuba. *Birth Defects Original Article Series* 28(3):52–57.

Hetzel BS, Maberly GF. 1986. Iodine. In Mertz (ed.). *Trace Elements in Human and Animal Nutrition* 2:139–208.

Hill K. 1999. Levels and trends in perinatal and neonatal mortality in developing countries. In *Reducing Perinatal and Neonatal Mortality: Report of a Meeting*. Baltimore, Maryland. May 10–12, 1999.

Hinman AR, Hersh BS, de Quadros CA. 1998. Rational use of rubella vaccine for prevention of congenital rubella syndrome in the Americas. *Pan American Journal of Public Health* 4(3):156–160.

Hinman AR, Irons B, Lewis M, Kandola K. 2002. Economic analyses of rubella and rubella vaccines: A global review. *Bulletin of the World Health Organization* 80(4):264–270.

Hitzeroth HW, Niehaus CE, Brill DC. 1995. Phenylketonuria in South Africa. A report on the status quo. *South African Medical Journal* 85(1):33–36.

Hogge JS, Hogge WA. 1996. Preconception genetic counseling. *Clinical Obstetrics and Gynecology* 39(4):751–762.

House H, McAlister M, Naidoo C. 1990. *Zimbabwe Steps Ahead*. Nottingham, UK: Catholic Institute for International Relations.

Immunization Working Group of the Mexico-United States Binational Commission. 2000. Measles, rubella, and congenital rubella syndrome—United States and Mexico, 1997–1999. *Morbidity and Mortality Weekly Report* 49(46):1048–1050, 1059.

International Labor Organization, United Nations Educational, Scientific and Cultural Organization, World Health Organization (ILO, UNESCO, WHO). 1994. *Community Based Rehabilitation for and with People with Disabilities*. Joint Position Paper. Geneva: World Health Organization.

Institute of Medicine (IOM). 1996. *Fetal Alcohol Syndrome: Diagnosis, Epidemiology, Prevention, and Treatment*. Washington, DC: National Academy Press.

Jaovisidha A, Ajjimarkorn S, Panburana P, Somboonsub O, Berabutya Y, Rungsiprakarn R. 2000. Prevention and control of thalassemia in Ramathibodi Hospital, Thailand. *Southeast Asian Journal of Tropical Medicine and Public Health* 31(3):561–565.

Jellis J. 1988. Taking orthopaedics to the people. *Bailliére's Clinical and Tropical Medicine Community Discussion* 3:257–263.

Jenkins T. 1990. Medical genetics in South Africa. *Journal of Medical Genetics* 27(12):760–779.

Jonsson T. 1994. OMAR in rehabilitation: *A Guide on Operations Monitoring and Results*. UNDP Interregional Programme for Disabled People. Geneva: United Nations Development Program.

Josefson D. 2001. Rubella vaccine may be safe in early pregnancy. *British Medical Journal* 322(7288):695.

Kale JS. 1999. Haemophilia: Scope for rehabilitation in India. *Journal of Postgraduate Medicine* 45(4):127.

Kaneko S, Battino D, Andermann E, Wada K, Kan R, Takeda A, Nakane Y, Ogawa Y, Avanzini G, Fumarola C, Granata T, Molteni F, Pardi G, Minotti L, Canger R, Dansky L, Oguni M, Lopes-Cendas I, Sherwin A, Andermann F, Seni MH, Okada M, Teranishi T. 1999. Congenital malformations due to antiepileptic drugs. *Epilepsy Research* 33(2–3):145–158.

Kate SL. 2001. Health problems of tribal population groups from the state of Maharashtra. *Indian Journal of Medical Sciences* 55(2):99–108.

Kavakli K, Nisli G, Aydinok Y, Oztop S, Cetingul N, Aydogdu S, Yalman O. 1997. Prophylactic therapy for hemophilia in a developing country, Turkey. *Pediatric Hematology and Oncology* 14(2):151–152, 158.

Keskin A, Turk T, Polat A, Koyuncu H, Saracoglu B. 2000. Premarital screening of beta-thalassemia trait in the province of Denizli, Turkey. *Acta Haematology* 104(1):31–33.

Kim NH, Park BM, Lee HM. 1990. Congenital dislocation of the hip—a long-term follow-up in Korea. *Yonsei Medical Journal* 31(2):134–143.

King RA, Hearing VJ, Creel DJ, Oetting WS. 1996. Abnormalities of pigmentation. In Emery AEH, Rimoin DL (eds.). *Emery and Rimoin's Principles and Practice of Medical Genetics*. New York: Churchill Livingstone. Pp. 1193–1194.

Kirklin JW, Barrat-Boyes BG (eds.). 1993. *Coarctation of the Aorta, and Interrupted Aortic Arch. Cardiac Surgery,* 2nd edition. Vol. 2. New York: Churchill Livingstone. P. 1274.

Koren A, Segal-Kupershmit D, Zalman L, Levin C, Abu Hana M, Palmor H, Luder A, Attias D. 1999. Effect of hydroxyurea in sickle cell anemia and sickle cell beta-thalassemia. *Pediatric Hematology and Oncology* 16(3):221–232.

Kromberg J. 1992. Albinism in the South African negro: IV. Attitudes and the death myth. *Birth Defects Original Article Series* 28(1):159–166.

Kyzer S. 1991. Congenital idiopathic clubfoot. *Orthopaedic Nursing* 10(4):11–18.

Leck I. 2000. Congenital dislocation of the hip. In Wald N, Leck I (eds.). 2000. *Antenatal and Neonatal Screening,* 2nd edition. New York: Oxford University Press. Pp. 398–424.

Lees CM, Davies S, Dezateux C. 2000. Neonatal screening for sickle cell disease. Cochrane Database System Review (2):CD0001913.

Li M, Qian QD, Qu CY, Liu DR, Zhang CD, Jia QZ, Wang HX, Zhang PY, Eastman CJ, Boyages SC, Maberly GF. 1989. A Survey of inland iodine excess goiter in Taiyuan suburbs and its immunological changes. *Journal of Chinese Endocrinology and Metabolism* 5:75–76.

Loukopoulos D. 1996. Current status of thalassemia and the sickle cell syndromes in Greece. *Seminars in Hematology* 33(1):76–86.

Lugovska R, Vevere P, Andrusaite R, Kornejeva A. 1999. Newborn screening for PKU and congenital hypothyroidism in Latvia. *Southeast Asian Journal of Tropical Medicine and Public Health* 30(suppl 2):52–53.

Lund PM. 1998. Living with albinism: A study of affected adults in Zimbabwe. *Journal of Social Biology and Human Affairs* 63:3–10.

Lund PM. 2001. Health and education of children with albinism in Zimbabwe. *Health Education and Research* 16(1):1–7.

Macri CN, de Gentile AS, Manterola A, Tomezzoli S, Reis FC, Garcia IL, Fernandez JLL. 1991. Epidemiology of cystic fibrosis in Latin America: Preliminary communication. *Pediatric Pulmonology* 10(4):250.

Mahashur AA. 1993. Cystic fibrosis. *Journal of Association of Physicians of India* 41(2):71–72.

Mariga L, Phachaka L. 1993. *Integrating Children with Special Education Needs into Regular Schools in Lesotho. Report of a Feasibility Study*. Lesotho: United Nations Children's Fund.

Massad E, Burattini MN, de Azevedo Neto RS, Yang HM, Coutinho FAB, Zanetta DMT. 1994. A model-based design of a vaccination strategy against rubella in a non-immunized community of São Paulo State, Brazil. *Epidemiology and Infection* 112:579–594.

Massad E, Azevedo-Neto RS, Burattini MN, Zanetta DM, Coutinho FA, Yang HM, Moraes JC, Pannuti CS, Souza VA, Silveira AS, Struchiner CJ, Oselka GW, Camargo MC, Omoto TM, Passos SD. 1995. Assessing the efficacy of a mixed vaccination strategy against rubella in São Paulo, Brazil. *International Journal of Epidemiology* 24(4):842–850.

McClendon JF. 1939. *Iodine and the incidence of goiter*. Minneapolis: University of Minnesota Press. Pp. 3–57.

McConachie H, Huq S, Munir S, Ferdous S, Zaman SS, Khan NZ. 2000. A randomized controlled trial of alternative modes of service provision for children with cerebral palsy in Bangladesh. *Journal of Pediatrics* 137(6):769–776.

McConkey R, O'Toole B. 1999. Towards the new millennium. In O'Toole B, McConkey R. (eds.). *Developing Countries for People with Disabilities*. Chorley, Lancashire, UK: Lisieux Hall Publications. P. 8.

McIntosh GC, Olshan AF, Baird PA. 1995. Paternal age and the risk of birth defects in offspring. *Epidemiology* 6(3):282–288.

McKay DW. 1982. New concept approach to clubfoot treatment. Section I. Principles and morbid anatomy. *Journal of Pediatric Orthopaedics*, 2, 347–356.

Medbø IU. 1961. Early diagnosis and treatment of the hip joint dysplasia. *Acta Orthopaedica Scandinavica* 31:282–315.

MEDLINEplus Medical Encyclopedia. 2001a. Cystic Fibrosis. Available online at www.nlm.nih.gov/medlineplus/ency/article/000107.htm.

MEDLINEplus Medical Encyclopedia. 2001b. Toxoplasmosis. Available online at www.nlm.nih.gov/medlineplus/ency/article/000637.htm.

Meloni T, Forteleoni G, Meloni GF. 1992. Marked decline of favism after neonatal glucose-6-phosphate dehydrogenase screening and health education: The northern Sardinian experience. *Acta Haematologica* 87(1–2):29–31.

Mendes DG, Roffman M. 1980. Early detection and treatment of congenital dislocation of the hip in the newborn. *Israel Journal of Medical Sciences* 16(4):247–249.

Modell B, Kuliev A. 1990. Changing paternal age distribution and the human mutation rate in Europe. *Human Genetics* 86(2):198–202.

Moos MK. 1994. *Preconceptional Health Promotion: March of Dimes Nursing Modules*. New York: March of Dimes Birth Defects Foundation.

MRC (Medical Research Council) Vitamin Study Research Group. 1991. Prevention of neural tube defects: Results of the Medical Research Council Vitamin Study. *Lancet* 338(8760):135.

Munir KM, Beardslee WR. 1999. Developmental psychiatry: Is there any other kind? *Harvard Review of Psychiatry* 6(5):250–262.

Nahmias AJ, Schwahn MG. 1985. Neonatal herpes simplex: A worldwide disease which is potentially preventable and treatable. *Progress in Clinical and Biological Research* 163B:355–362.

Oakley GP. 1993. Folic acid-preventable spina bifida and anencephaly (editorial). *Journal of the American Medical Association* 269(10):1292–1293.

Oakley GP Jr. 2002a. Inertia on folic acid fortification: Public health malpractice. *Teratology* 66(1):44–54.

Oakley GP Jr. 2002b. Delaying folic acid fortification of flour. *British Medical Journal* 324(7350):1348–1349.

Operation Smile. 2001. Available online at http://www.operationsmile.org.

Ounap K, Lillevali H, Metspalu A, Lipping-Sitska M. 1998. Development of the phenylketonuria screening programme in Estonia. *Journal of Medical Screening* 5(1):22–23.

Parekh PK. 1985. Prevalence and management of congenital club-feet (talipes equinobarus) in Zambia. *East African Medical Journal* 62(1):38–47.

Perry KR, Brown DW, Parry JV, Panday S, Pipkin C, Richards A. 1993. The detection of measles, mumps, and rubella antibodies in saliva using antibody capture radioimmunoassays. *Journal of Medical Virology* 40(3):235–240.

Pilu G, Reece E, Romero R, Bovicelli L, Hobbins J. 1986. Prenatal diagnosis of craniofacial malformations with ultrasonography. *American Journal of Obstetrics and Gynecology* 155(1):45–50.

Plotkin SA, Katz M, Cordero JF. 1999. The eradication of rubella. *Journal of the American Medical Association* 281(6):561–562.

Porter RW. 1987. Congenital talipes equinovarus: II. A staged method of surgical management. *Journal of Bone and Joint Surgery* 69(5):826–831.

Poustie VJ, Rutherford P. 2001. Dietary interventions for phenylketonuria. *Cochrane Database of Systematic Reviews*, Issue 2.

Powell G. 2000. *Report on Childhood Disability in Sub-Saharan Africa.* Harare: Department of Pediatrics and Child Health, University of Zimbabwe Medical School.

Rabbi-Bortolini E, Bernardino AL, Lopes AL, Ferri AS, Passos-Bueno MR, Zatz M. 1998. Sweat electrolyte and cystic fibrosis mutation analysis allows early diagnosis in Brazilian children with clinical signs compatible with cystic fibrosis. *American Journal of Medical Genetics* 76(4):288–290.

Ramalingaswami V. 2000. The public health imperative of permanent elimination of iodine deficiency. In Geertman RM (ed.). *Eighth World Salt Symposium.* Vol. 1. Amsterdam: Elsevier. Pp. 3–11.

Ramsey PL, Lasser S, MacEwen GD. 1976. Congenital dislocation of the hip. Use of the Pavlik harness in the child during the first six months of life. *Journal of Bone and Joint Surgery* 58(7):1000.

Rao RS, Chakladar BK, Nair NS, Kutty PR, Acharya D, Bhat V, Chandrasekhar S, Rodrigues VC, Kumar P, Nagaraj K, Prasad KN, Krishnan L. 1996. Influence of parental literacy and socio-economic status on infant mortality. *Indian Journal of Pediatrics* 63(6):795–800.

Robertson SE, Cutts FT, Samuel R, Diaz-Ortega JL. 1997. Control of rubella and congenital rubella syndrome (CRS) in developing countries, Part 2: Vaccination against rubella. *Bulletin of the World Health Organization* 75(1):69–80.

Rodriguez L, Sanchez R, Hernandez J, Carrillo L, Oliva J, Heredero L. 1997. Results of 12 years' combined maternal serum alpha-fetoprotein screening and ultrasound fetal monitoring for prenatal detection of fetal malformations in Havana City, Cuba. *Prenatal Diagnosis* 17(4):301–304.

Ross HL, Elias S. 1997. Maternal serum screening for fetal genetic disorders. *Obstetrics and Gynecology Clinics in North America* 24(1):33–47.

Rygg IH, Olesen K, Boesen I. 1971. The life history of teratology of Fallot. *Danish Medical Bulletin* 18(suppl 2):25–30.

Saborio M. 1992. Experience in providing genetic services in Costa Rica. *Birth Defects Original Article Series* 28(3):96–102.

Scott R, Evans S. 1997. Non-specialist management of tropical talipes. *Tropical Doctor* 27(1):22–25.

Sengupta A. 1987. The management of congenital talipes equinovarus in developing countries. *International Orthopaedics* 11(3):183–187.

Simpson JL, Golbus MS. 1992. Spectrum of autosomal chromosome abnormalities. In *Genetics in Obstetrics and Gynecology,* 2nd edition. Philadelphia: W.B. Saunders Co. Pp. 53–59, 61–78, 207.

Sinha SN. 1987. A simple guide to management of club foot. *Papua New Guinea Medical Journal* 30(2):165–168.

Smith HW, Keen M, Edwards E. 1991. Cleft lip and palate surgery in La Ceiba, Honduras. *Archives of Otolaryngology—Head and Neck Surgery* 117(12):1356–1359.

Stanbury JB. 1998. Prevention of iodine deficiency. In Howson CP, Kennedy ET, Horowitz A. (eds.). *Prevention of Micronutrient Deficiencies: Tools for Policymakers and Public Health Workers.* Washington, DC: National Academy Press. Pp. 177–179.

Steensma DP, Hoyer JD, Fairbanks VF. 2001. Hereditary red blood cell disorders in Middle Eastern patients. *Mayo Clinic Proceedings* 76(3):285–293.

Stolk EA, Post HA, Rutten FF, Molenaar JC, Busschbach JJ. 2000. Cost-effectiveness of neonatal surgery: A review. *Journal of Pediatric Surgery* 35(4):588–592.

Thorburn MJ. 1993. Recent developments in low-cost screening and assessment of childhood disabilities in Jamaica. Part I: Screening. *West Indian Medical Journal* 42(1):10–20.

Thorburn MJ. 2000. Training of CBR personnel: Current issues and future trends. *Asia Pacific Disability Rehabilitation Journal* 11:12–17.

Thorburn M, Desai P, Paul TJ, Malcolm L, Durkin M, Davidson L. 1992. Identification of childhood disability in Jamaica: The ten question screen. *International Journal of Rehabilitation Research* 15(2):115–127.

Thorburn MJ, Paul TJ, Malcolm LM. 1993. Recent developments in low-cost screening and assessment of childhood disabilities in Jamaica. Part 2: Assessment. *West Indian Medical Journal* 42(2):46–52.

Tookey PA, Jones G, Miller BH, Peckham CS. 1991. Rubella vaccination in pregnancy. *Communicable Disease Report* (London:Review) 1(8):R86–R88.

Turco VT. 1974. Discussion. *Orthopedic Clinics of North America* 5(1):58.

United Nations Educational, Scientific and Cultural Organization (UNESCO) and the Ministry of Education and Science, Spain. 1994. *The Salamanca Statement. The Final Report of the World Conference on Special Needs Education, Access and Quality.* Paris.

United Nations Children's Fund (UNICEF). 2000a. *Ending Iodine Deficiency Forever: A Goal Within Our Grasp.* New York: United Nations Children's Fund and the World Health Organization.

United Nations Children's Fund (UNICEF). 2000b. *The State of the World's Children 2001.* New York: United Nations Children's Fund.

U.S. Food and Drug Administration. 1996. Food standards: Amendment of standards of identity for enriched grain products to require addition of folic acid. *Federal Register* 61(44):8781–8807.

Vanderpas JB, Contempre B, Duale NL, Deckx H, Bebe N, Longombe AO, Thilly CH, Diplock AT, Dumont JE. 1993. Selenium deficiency mitigates hypothyroxinemia in iodine-deficient subjects. *American Journal of Clinical Nutrition* 57(2 suppl):271S–275S.

van Ginneken JK, Lob-Levyt J, Gove S. 1996. Potential interventions for preventing pneumonia among young children in developing countries: Promoting maternal education. *Tropical Medicine and International Health* 1(3):283–294.

Verjee ZH. 1993. Glucose 6-phosphate dehydrogenase deficiency in Africa—review. *East African Medical Journal* 70(4 suppl):40, 42–43.

Vichinsky EP, Styles LA, Colangelo LH, Wright EC, Castro O, Nickerson B. 1997. Cooperative Study of Sickle Cell Disease. Acute chest syndrome in sickle cell disease: Clinical presentation and course. *Blood* 89(5):1787–1792.

Viljoen D.1999. Fetal alcohol syndrome. *South African Medical Journal* 89(9):958–960.

Wald NJ, Hackshaw AK. 2000. Advances in antenatal screening for Down syndrome. *Best Practice and Research in Clinical Obstetrics and Gynecology* 14(4):543–551, 563–580.

Wald N, Leck I, Gray JAM. 2000. Ethics of antenatal and neonatal screening. In Wald N, Leck I (eds.). *Antenatal and Neonatal Screening,* 2nd edition. New York: Oxford University Press. Pp. 543–555.

Wald NJ, Huttly WJ, Hackshaw AK. 2003. Antenatal screening for Down's syndrome with the quadruple test. *Lancet* 361(9360):835–838.

Wallace M, Hurwitz B. 1998. Preconception care: Who needs it, who wants it, and how should it be provided? *British Journal of General Practice* 48:963–966.

Weatherall D, Letsky EA. 2000. Genetic haematological disorders. In Wald N, Leck I (eds.). *Antenatal and neonatal screening,* 2nd edition. New York: Oxford University Press. Pp. 260–261.

Werner D. 1987. *Disabled Village Children.* Palo Alto, CA: Hesperian Foundation.

World Bank. 1993. *World Development Report 1993: Investing in Health.* New York: World Bank.

World Health Organization (WHO). 1980. *International Classification of Impairments, Disabilities and Handicaps.* Geneva: WHO.

World Health Organization (WHO). 1985. *Community Approaches to the Control of Hereditary Diseases.* Geneva: WHO.

World Health Organization (WHO). 1993. *Promoting the Development of Young Children with Cerebral Palsy: A Guide for Mid-Level Rehabilitation Workers.* Geneva: WHO.

World Health Organization (WHO). 1996a. *Control of Hereditary Diseases: Report of a WHO Scientific Working Group.* WHO Technical Report Series. Geneva: WHO.

World Health Organization (WHO). 1996b. *Recommended Iodine Levels in Salt and Guidelines for Monitoring their Adequacy and Effectiveness.* Geneva: WHO/UNICEF/ICCIDD.

World Health Organization (WHO). 1997. Human genetics. Proposed International Guidelines on Ethical Issues in Medical Genetics and Genetic Services. Available online at http://www.who.int/ncd/hgn/hgnethic.htm.

World Health Organization (WHO). 1999. *Human Genetics: Services for the Prevention and Management of Genetic Disorders and Birth Defects in Developing Countries: Report of a Joint WHO/WOAPBD Meeting.* Geneva: WHO.

World Health Organization (WHO). 2000a. *Primary Health Care Approaches for the Prevention and Control of Congenital Genetic Disorders: Report of a WHO Meeting.*

World Health Organization (WHO). 2000b. Preventing congenital rubella syndrome. *Weekly Epidemiology Record* 75(36):290–295.

World Health Organization (WHO). 2001. *Assessment of Iodine Deficiency Disorders and Monitoring Their Elimination. A Guide for Program Managers,* 2nd edition. Geneva: WHO. Pp. 1–122.

World Health Organization, United Nations Children's Fund, International Council for the Control of Iodine Deficiency Disorders (WHO, UNICEF, ICCIDD). 1999. Progress towards elimination of iodine deficiency disorders. Geneva: WHO (unpublished document) WHO/NHD/99.4.

Yang YH, Ju KS, Kim SB, Cho YH, Lee JH, Lee SH, Choi OH, Chun JH, Kim JI, Kim HJ, Sohn YS. 1999. The Korean Collaborative Study on 11,000 prenatal genetic amniocentesis. *Yonsei Medical Journal* 40(5):460–466.

Zaman SS, Khan NZ, Islam S (eds.). 1996. *From Awareness to Action: Ensuring Health, Education and Rights of Disabled.* Dhaka: Bangladesh Protibondhi Foundation.

Zar HJ, Bateman E, Ramsay M. 1998. New advances in cystic fibrosis—implications for developing countries. *South African Medical Journal* 88(8):968.

Zimbabwe Ministry of Education, Sports and Culture. 1998. *School Psychological Services and Special Needs Education.* Annual Report.

4

Incorporating Care for Birth Defects into Health Care Systems

ealth care systems and the services they provide vary widely among, and even within, countries. National and local priorities, infrastructure, and financial and human resources each play a role in determining the extent and speed with which interventions addressing birth defects can be incorporated into primary care and thus made widely available. This chapter describes strategies for introducing interventions for the prevention and care of birth defects into health care systems in developing countries, the coordination of these strategies at the national level, and the building of infrastructure to support and strengthen reproductive health care and reduce the impact of birth defects.

STRATEGIES FOR ADDRESSING BIRTH DEFECTS

Several low-cost preventive strategies for reducing the impact of birth defects, described in Chapter 3 and summarized in Table 4-1, can be made widely available through community health programs. This section describes the steps to achieve this goal, also care for children who have birth defects, and, for countries that have been successful in lowering infant mortality through effective health care services, the introduction of genetic screening and diagnosis for common and severe birth defects.

Enhancing Current Reproductive Health Services

Primary health care in almost all settings includes maternal and child health (MCH) services, which include reproductive health. The services

122

TABLE 4-1 Interventions to Reduce the Impact of Birth Defects

Program Area	Risk Factors To Be Addressed Before and During Pregnancy	Interventions
Reproductive health care and family planning	Unwanted births Pregnancy in women over 35 Preexisting maternal diseases	Family planning information Education for couples on birth defects Neonatal care
Micronutrient deficiencies	Iodine Folic acid	Universal access to iodized salt Fortification of staple food with folic acid
Exposure to teratogens	Rubella Alcohol use Teratogenic medications Environmental teratogens	Vaccination Public health messages and counseling on limiting or avoiding alcohol use and avoiding teratogenic medications and environmental teratogens Regulations on environmental teratogens

themselves vary with the needs and resources of the community and with the level of access to secondary and tertiary care for more complex and difficult health conditions.

Primary, secondary, and tertiary care

Primary care is provided at the local level. There are very few nurses and physicians in most developing countries (see Figures 4-1 and 4-2), and most of them practice in urban settings. The majority of people receive care at community health centers served by nonspecialized health workers or by nurses or physicians linked to specialist resources at secondary and tertiary health centers. The introduction or expansion of prevention and care for birth defects in developing countries is best undertaken in primary health care facilities. Although primary care providers may have rudimentary training and few medications or diagnostic tools, they can nonetheless provide important preventive services, such as family planning, information on the causes of birth defects, micronutrient supplements, immunization, and guidance on avoiding teratogens. By forging strong linkages with secondary, tertiary, and national health care centers and by collaborating with nongovernmental organizations (NGOs) and international agencies, primary care services can increase their ability to address birth defects within communities.

Secondary care is provided in district or regional hospitals, which are staffed by general physicians, medical technicians, and nurses. These facilities

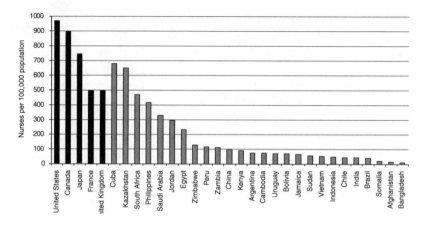

FIGURE 4-1   Number of nurses per 100,000 population in selected countries. Black bars represent developed countries. Gray bars represent developing countries.
SOURCE: World Health Organization, 1998a.

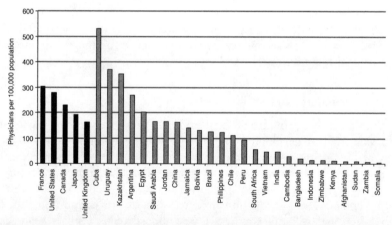

FIGURE 4-2   Number of physicians per 100,000 population in selected countries, 1990–1998. Black bars represent developed countries. Gray bars represent developing countries.
SOURCE: World Health Organization, 1998a.

can treat more severe and complex medical conditions and provide routine surgery; they also have access to diagnostic equipment and laboratory facilities. District hospitals can expand the services offered at primary care centers by providing essential medications and vaccinations on-site and by using mobile care teams. Medical professionals from secondary facilities can support and train community health care workers, make regular visits to primary care centers to monitor their reproductive health care, review more difficult cases, and assist in identifying patients in need of referral. Training of community health workers can include, along with the care of other conditions, instruction on the prevention of birth defects, counseling and recording of family histories, and identification of patients requiring referral.

Tertiary care, the most specialized health care, is provided in larger, urban hospitals. Because health care resources are limited and the operating costs of tertiary centers are high, these facilities are limited in number in developing countries. As part of reproductive care for patients referred from primary care centers, tertiary care hospitals can provide genetic screening (preconceptional, prenatal, and postnatal) and surgery to correct certain birth defects. Tertiary care centers can also serve as facilities for collecting epidemiological data, providing staff training, creating and distributing educational health materials, and conducting clinical and operational research (World Health Organization, 1999).

Support of primary and secondary health care facilities by tertiary centers can contribute to the development and maintenance of affordable, good-quality health care. Studies conducted at tertiary centers can identify common birth defects and their risk factors, also preventive strategies, and effective treatment and rehabilitation. Most important is the evidence base for determining national health priorities and community health care services. Moreover, training curricula developed at these facilities can be adapted for staff at secondary and primary care levels (Lansang and Olveda, 1994).

Capacity for expanded services

Provision of comprehensive preventive and therapeutic care for birth defects is a long-term goal for most countries. However, the low-cost preventive strategies recommended in this report warrant immediate evaluation and incorporation into primary care services. Continuing progress toward comprehensive services can be achieved through an iterative process that involves introducing an intervention that has been proven affordable and effective in a similar setting, then evaluating and improving its effectiveness in the local setting—all with support and oversight from secondary and tertiary centers. Involving the relevant nonhealth sectors—education, social services, industry, and environment—in the development of interventions can advance progress toward common goals. International organizations can also assist countries in the implementation of cost-effective programs.

Laboratory standards

The diagnosis of most genetic disorders and birth defects requires specialized tests. Because specimens are generally processed in regional laboratories to maintain quality and cost control, systems are needed for the transportation of specimens from primary and secondary health centers to tertiary health centers (World Health Organization, 1999). Laboratory staff should be accredited, and facilities and performance monitored, in order to maintain accurate, reliable diagnostic services. Standardization of laboratory tests requires external quality assessment, training, and education (Bunyaratvej, 1999).

Training

Development of staff expertise and provision of ongoing training are essential to improving reproductive health care. The framework for training, as for specific interventions themselves, should be based on evidence of proven effectiveness and affordability. Important areas for training include clinical practice or treatment, epidemiology, counseling, rehabilitation, and operational research.

Collaborations

Alliances between public health care providers and private physicians, educators, community organizations, community-based NGOs, and rehabilitation programs can improve the effectiveness of interventions in reducing the impact of birth defects.

Private Physicians. Health care services in several Latin American countries and in India have been privatized over the last two decades, so that much of primary care in these countries takes place in the private sector. In India, for example, private physicians provide about half of all primary care and as much as 80 percent in some states. Even the rural and urban poor consult private physicians because they are accessible, charge a relatively low consultation fee, and are widely perceived as providing better care than the public health system (Chisholm et al., 2000).

Educators. Health education has been incorporated into many school curricula. This should include instruction on reproductive health and well-being and the locally relevant risks for birth defects.

Community Organizations. Although relatively few and often poorly funded, community organizations can facilitate mutual support and sharing of experience among patients, families, and caregivers. NGOs and parent groups can together establish facilities such as vocational training centers, day care centers, and supported-living facilities staffed by community volunteers. By educating the community about birth defects, these local groups can change negative attitudes and draw the attention of policy makers to the needs of affected individuals and their families.

NGOs. For several community-based NGOs, health care services are part of a broad development agenda. These organizations are found most commonly in less developed regions that tend to be underserved by government-provided health care services, such as India and sub-Saharan Africa.

Community-Based Rehabilitation (CBR) Programs. These low-cost programs coordinate medical guidance and community resources in the rehabilitation of children and adults disabled by birth defects, allowing them to live as normally as possible (see Chapter 3). Some of the most successful CBR programs are able to mainstream disabled children into public education at the earliest opportunity and assist them in the transition from school to employment. In addition to providing long-term care and support for patients and their families, CBR addresses the isolation and stigma often experienced by disabled persons. These programs can be linked to and supported by institutional and hospital-based programs to create a comprehensive rehabilitation service.

International Partnerships. Building the capacity of developing countries to provide strong reproductive health care requires international contributions of expertise and resources. Two kinds of international partnership that can be especially effective are professional societies and international organizations.

The international community of health care professionals can advocate that birth defects receive attention from health policy makers commensurate with the contribution of the disorders to the overall burden of disease. Such attention is particularly important for conditions that result in stigmatization. Professional societies can provide a realistic perspective to policy makers—who are often reluctant to provide treatment and rehabilitation to patients unless they perceive an economic return to the community—and can assist them in developing cost-effective health care policies.

WHO has supported the implementation of interventions to reduce the impact of birth defects in developing countries, proposed guidelines for genetic services, and addressed ethical issues arising from genetic services (World Health Organization, 1998b, 1999, 2001). The United Nations Children's Fund (UNICEF) and the United Nations Development Programme have supported vaccination and other programs for the control of infectious diseases. Both organizations could also take an active role in reproductive health and the reduction of birth defects. Save the Children has initiated a global program on reproductive health in developing countries. The World Bank and other development banks also have active programs on reproductive health. In addition, the World Bank fostered development of the disability-adjusted life years (DALY) measure and the estimation of disease burden in the Global Burden of Disease Study (World Bank, 1993). This frontier could be further advanced with efforts to better estimate the disease burden of birth defects among children in developing countries, an area in which the evidence base is particularly limited. The March of Dimes has coordinated professional organizations in the development of international databases on birth defects, supported research, and has educated families and the general public on these disorders.

To meet broad needs for family planning and other reproductive health measures, child survival, and HIV/AIDS care, five private voluntary organizations—ADRA (Adventit Development Relief Agency), CARE (Cooperative for Assistance and Relief Everywhere), PATH (Program for Appropriate Technology in Health), Plan International, and Save the Children—have NGO Networks for Health. This consortium aims to improve health information and services in specific developing countries (Ashman, 2001). The Population and Family Planning Expansion Project, implemented by CARE and funded by the U.S. Agency for International Development, supports capacity building for family planning and reproductive health care. Initial projects combined community-based services with links to secondary and tertiary facilities to improve access to health care in difficult-to-reach rural and periurban communities. The project also provides training for health care workers in contraceptive technology and counseling skills and for managers in enhancing supervisory, monitoring, and evaluative skills (Cooperative for Assistance and Relief Everywhere, 1999; Wilcox, 1999).

Launching Public Health Campaigns

An important component of some interventions involves education and public health messages on such issues as:

- The importance of family planning,
- Prevention of unplanned births for all women and for those over 35 years of age,
- Awareness of the increased risk of birth defects in consanguineous unions,
- Prevention of iodine deficiency,
- The need for folic acid supplementation,
- Limited use or avoidance of alcohol consumption during pregnancy,
- Avoidance of exposure to teratogenic medications and pollutants, and
- Control of rubella and other infectious diseases.

Such public health campaigns can employ radio and television messages and informational pamphlets. Important risks may also be addressed through plays and films that portray the avoidance of risky behaviors (Mohammed, 2001).

Introducing Genetic Services

Once a country has reduced infant mortality rates by incorporating the most cost-effective interventions into health care programs, there are guidelines for evaluating its capacity and readiness to implement a genetic screening and counseling program (World Health Organization, 2000a). Should such a program be found appropriate, the next step is to determine the locally important conditions to be screened and appropriate screening procedures, so that accurate, reliable, and cost-effective services can be provided. Genetic screening programs should be developed through a logical, orderly approach consistent with available resources, staff training and experience, the capability for diagnostic follow-up of those identified to be at high risk for a disorder, and the capacity of staff trained for counseling. Staff in primary care centers can identify patients to be screened or referred. Secondary and tertiary centers can provide genetic screening and counseling and, where necessary, follow-up diagnoses and treatment. The number of centers with the capacity for genetic screening will depend on the balance between accessibility of services and provision of equitable, cost-effective services for all segments of a population.

In countries where there is an unusually high occurrence of certain genetic disorders, public programs can provide preconceptional screening to identify carriers, prenatal screening to detect fetal disorders, and early neonatal screening for high-risk pregnancies. Countries that support screening for specific birth defects include Cuba, Iran, and South Africa. In many other countries, genetic screening is limited to middle- and high–income patients with access to private medical practices. Finally, to be successful, genetic screening programs must be supported and championed by political and religious leaders and maintained through strong commitment by national and local health departments.

NATIONAL POLICY AND LEADERSHIP

National public health policy should address preventable risk factors for birth defects, some of which are more common in developing than in developed countries (see Chapter 2). National governments can lead efforts to identify and strengthen interventions that protect against these disorders.

Strategies for Intervention

When an effective program of primary care is in place, even in resource-poor countries, it can be expanded successfully to incorporate additional interventions (including, where appropriate, genetic screening) into basic reproductive care. Incorporating these interventions will, however, involve governments in decisions concerning budget priorities. Most important to this process will be having accurate data on the prevalence and disease burden of specific birth defects and on the cost-effectiveness of interventions that are under way in comparable settings (discussed in detail in Chapter 3).

The specific interventions recommended in Chapter 3 that deserve universal implementation include family planning, dietary supplementation with iodine and folic acid, control of infectious diseases, and avoidance of teratogens during pregnancy. Information on locally relevant teratogenic medications to be avoided should be conveyed to primary care providers, as well as to the general public; governments may also consider limiting access to teratogenic medications such as thalidomide. Exposure to mercury and other terogenic pollutants can be reduced through collaborations between health departments and other government agencies to develop legislation on environmental protection and occupational hazards.

Increased availability of genetic screening is likely to raise ethical issues that require resolution at the national level. The agreement reached on ethical dilemmas will vary with the social, religious, and legal traditions of each country and with the capacity of the health care system.

Comprehensive programs that include prevention, treatment, and rehabilitation of birth defects can be costly (Waitzman et al., 1994). However, where political will is strong, as in the example of thalassemia prevention and treatment in Iran (see Box 3-9), impressive gains can be made in addressing birth defects with cost-effective interventions. Accurate epidemiological data and parental concern about thalassemia in Iran created a national awareness of the societal burden caused by the disorder. Policy makers recognized the need for treatment and introduced it. The high cost of treatment then led to more affordable genetic screening and prevention of thalassemia (Angastiniotis et al., 1995; World Health Organization, 2000b).

Public education on the causes, impact, and prevention of birth defects deserves the support of both government agencies and NGOs and can be provided through patient and family support groups and school-based initiatives. National and international alliances of people with birth defects and their families provide valuable support and education for their members, health professionals, and the public (World Health Organization, 1999).

Coordination of Services

A key role for governments is coordinating the care provided by different tiers of the health care system. Support and oversight of primary care must be emphasized, along with connections to secondary and tertiary care through physicians and specialists at district and national facilities. Policies should be established to guide the progress of patients along established pathways as they seek genetic screening, surgery, or other advanced care.

Although each community should define its own health care priorities, national policy can support this process by establishing a national program of basic reproductive care. Such a program should set uniform standards for training and performance; collect and interpret surveillance data; and establish networks of communication among health care providers, researchers, and policy makers.

Priority setting

National and local initiatives should be based on cost-effective interventions. Since prevention is the most affordable and effective strategy for addressing birth defects, community health workers should be trained in the importance of educating young people, and women in particular, on nutritional, infectious, teratogenic, and genetic risks. Likewise, health care policies that target common, severe birth defects in a community make the most efficient use of limited resources.

Training

Governments should establish standards for the training of personnel at all levels of health care to build a strong foundation for the primary care system. National training policies should also reflect the importance of continuing professional education for primary caregivers. Although training may be organized by local health services, it can be encouraged through national policies that make available such resources as quality instruction, distance learning, lectures, workshops, and access to journals and the Internet. The need to reduce the impact of birth defects should be addressed in the training of professionals, including physicians, nurses, and technicians.

Monitoring of health care delivery and outcomes

Surveillance of birth defects and related control programs, including data collected in primary care settings, provides the evidence base for evaluating the efficacy of current care and practice. National policy should therefore support the collection, analysis, and dissemination of information on health care outcomes (Lorenzo, 1994).

Internet communication

As resources can be made available, a central internet site can be established to serve as a repository of information on reproductive health, child health, and birth defects. This gateway site can enlist the participation of professionals, public health organizations, and advocates worldwide. It can include recent findings from surveillance and operational research; standardized versions of basic reproductive care, genetic screening and diagnosis, and therapeutic services for common birth defects in different settings; evaluation of interventions for cost-effectiveness; and access to training packages for distance learning. The site can also facilitate communication among health care providers, researchers, and policy makers at national centers and in the communities they serve.

Research

A robust agenda of epidemiological and operational research is needed to inform and support primary care interventions aimed at reducing neonatal mortality and morbidity due to birth defects (see Chapter 3). Research in the following areas should be given high priority:

• Epidemiological studies to measure the prevalence and burden of disease caused by common and severe birth defects in national and local settings. Even where financial resources are limited, this basic information provides the evidence base for decisions involving the potential impact and cost of specific interventions.
• Development of affordable surveillance and information systems for birth defects and evaluation of their reliability, validity, and feasibility.
• Rigorous evaluation of the effectiveness in local settings of interventions proven clinically- and cost-effective in similar settings in the prevention and treatment of birth defects. Preconceptional, prenatal, and neonatal screening might also be evaluated in programs that target specific prevalent, severe, and treatable birth defects. In addition, operational research should evaluate affordable, effective strategies for rehabilitation of children with birth defects in low-resource settings.
• Studies of the impact of health education programs for teenagers and young adults in terms of their awareness of the risk factors for birth defects, and on their behavior changes for a health pregnancy.
• Studies of the long-term health and psychosocial impact of birth defects.

Establishment of an operational research capacity can strongly support the planning and management of health care including reproductive health and reduction of the impact of birth defects. This is accomplished by providing the data needed for setting priorities among health problems, for justifying a focus on health care, and for evaluating interventions for their effectiveness (Morrow and Lansang, 1991). Research programs could also promote the development of an international cadre of professionals focused on these issues in developing countries. Successful models for such a research program are the Fogarty International Center Training and Research Programs at the U.S. National Institutes of Health, the WHO Special Programme for Research and Training in Tropical Diseases, and the program on reproductive health initiated recently at Save the Children. Collaboration on research associated with birth defects can be undertaken with a number of organizations in developed countries. National and local programs focused on reproductive health care and specific birth defects can increase the capacity for health research.

Two principal means of collecting epidemiological data for health care planning purposes are surveys and record keeping at the primary care level. In addition to surveys of the prevalence of specific birth defects among the general population, studies that attempt to describe how people seek family planning assistance or how patients with birth defects make use of different kinds of health care providers could be useful. Research on pathways to health care can identify areas for improvement in the efficiency of treatment and referral in health care systems. Programs such as the International Clinical Epidemiology Network strengthen epidemiological research skills.

CONCLUSION

Birth defects are an important and as yet poorly measured burden of disease in developing countries, but their burden on individuals is clear: the impact of birth defects is often severe, lifelong, demanding of a high level of care, and responsible for a substantial loss in quality of life for the patient and frequently the family as well. Epidemiological studies have provided some basic knowledge about birth defects in developing countries, including evidence of relatively high population prevalences, the contribution of various causes, and prospects for prevention. While the data are, on the whole, extremely limited, a variety of genetic, nutritional, infectious, and teratogenic causes are known. Many of these causes are preventable, and treatments can correct or reduce the impact of some birth defects, as can a variety of interventions involving education and rehabilitation. Nonetheless, few resources are devoted to programs to prevent birth defects or treat children with birth defects in low-income countries. The need to reduce birth defects in the developing world calls for innovative and sustained public health efforts and financial commitments.

REFERENCES

Angastiniotis M, Modell B, Englezos P, Boulyjenkov V. 1995. Prevention and control of haemoglobinopathies. *Bulletin of the World Health Organization* 73(3):375–386.

Ashman D. 2001. NGO Networks for Health Project. The partnerships at the global level among ADRA, CARE, PATH, PLAN International, and Save the Children in NGO Networks for Health. Available online at: www.ngonetworks.org.

Bunyaratvej A. 1999. Plan and process for hematology laboratory standard in Thailand. *Southeast Asian Journal of Tropical Medicine and Public Health* 30(suppl 3):173–174.

CARE. 1999. Final report of the Population and Family Planning Expansion (PFPE) Project. December. Available online at: www.ngonetworks.org.

Chisholm D, Sekar K, Kumar KK, Saeed K, James S, Mubbashar M, Murthy RS. 2000. Integration of mental health care into primary care. Demonstration cost–outcomes in India and Pakistan. *British Journal of Psychiatry* 176:581–588.

Lansang M, Olveda R. 1994. Institutional linkages: Strategic bridges for research capacity strengthening. *Acta Tropica* 57(2–3):139–145.

Lorenzo T. 1994. The identification of continuing education needs for community rehabilitation workers in a rural health district in the Republic of South Africa. *International Journal of Rehabilitation* Research 17(3):241–250.

Mohammed S. 2001. Personal communication networks and the effects of an entertainment-education radio soap opera in Tanzania. *Journal of Health Communication* 6(2):137–154.

Morrow RH, Lansang MA. 1991. The role of clinical epidemiology in establishing essential national health research capabilities in developing countries. *Infectious Disease Clinics of North America* 5(2):235–246.

Waitzman NJ, Romano PS, Scheffler RM. 1994. Estimates of the economic costs of birth defects. *Inquiry* 31(2):188–205.

Wilcox S. 1999. NGO Networks for Health Project. The story of CARE's successful integration of family planning and reproductive health services. February. Available online at: http://www.ngonetworks.org.

World Bank. 1993. *World Development Report 1993: Investing In Health*. New York: Oxford University Press.

World Health Organization (WHO). 1998a. WHO Estimates of Health Personnel: Physicians, Nurses, Midwives, Dentists and Pharmacists (around 1998). Available online at: http://www3.who.int/whosis/health_personnel/health_personnel.cfm?path=whosis, health_ personnel&language=english.

World Health Organization (WHO). 1998b. *Proposed International Guidelines on Ethical Issues in Medical Genetic and Genetic Services*. Geneva: WHO.

World Health Organization (WHO). 1999. *Human Genetics: Services for the Prevention and Management of Genetic Disorders and Birth Defects in Developing Countries*. Report of a Joint WHO/WOAPBD Meeting. Geneva: WHO.

World Health Organization (WHO). 2000a. *Primary Health Care Approaches for the Prevention and Control of Congenital Genetic Disorders: Report of a WHO Meeting*. Geneva: WHO.

World Health Organization (WHO). 2000b. The Special Programme for Research Training in Tropical Diseases. Available online at: http://www.who.int/tdr/.

World Health Organization (WHO). 2001. WHO estimates of health personnel. Available online at: http://who.int.org.

Appendix A

Prevalence of Birth Defects

The tables that follow address the prevalence of birth defects in a range of settings.

A-1   Birth defects
A-2   Down syndrome
A-3   Thalassemia
A-4   Sickle cell disease
A-5   Glucose-6-phosphate dehydrogenase deficiency
A-6   Oculocutaneous albinism
A-7   Cystic fibrosis
A-8   Phenylketonuria
A-9   Neural tube defects and hydrocephalus
A-10   Congenital heart disease
A-11   Cleft lip and/or cleft palate
A-12   Talipes
A-13   Developmental dysplasia of the hip

Many of the observed differences in the prevalence rates observed in different studies may be the result of different methodological approaches.

135

TABLE A-1   Studies on the Prevalence of Birth Defects

Country	Year	Population
Africa		
South Africa	1989–1992	Live births, Mankweng Hospital, Sovenga, Northern Transvaal ($n = 7,617$)
South Africa	1986–1989	Live births, Kalafong Hospital, Pretoria ($n = 17,351$)
Tunisia	1983–1984	Births, Wassila Bourgiba Hospital, Tunis (live births 9662, stillbirths 238) ($n = 10,000$)
Zimbabwe	1983	Births, Greater Harare Obstetric Unit, Harare ($n = 45,343$) 1
Uganda	1956–1957	Births, Mulago Hospital, Kampala (live births 1927, stillbirths 141) ($n = 2,068$)
Asia		
Malaysia	1984–1987	Live births, Alor Setar General Hospital ($n = 19,769$)
China	1988–1991	Births, National Center for Birth Defects Monitoring ($n = 2,750,588$)
Indonesia	1983–1987	Births, Gunung Wenang Hospital Manado, Jakarta ($n = 13,354$)

Method	Prevalence	Reference
Physical examination within 24 hours of birth Tests used to confirm clinically suspected cases: Biological specimens Radiographs Genetic reference Extrapolation, age 1 yr Extrapolation, age 5 yr	15/1,000 live births (major) 30.7/1,000 live births (major and minor) 37.4/1,000 57.1/1,000	Venter et al., 1995
Physical examination within 24 hours of birth	11.9/1,000 live births	Delport et al., 1995
Physical examination within 24 hours of birth Test used to confirm clinically suspected cases: Roentgenograms	24.8/1,000 births (major) 39.6/1,000 (major and minor)	Khrouf et al., 1986
Physical examination	2.1/1,000 births (major)	Crowther and Glyn-Jones, 1986
Physical examination at birth	18.9/1,000 births (major) 54/1,000 births (major and minor)	Simpkiss and Lowe, 1961
Physical examination within 48 hours of birth Tests used to confirm clinically suspected cases: Lab investigations Ultrasound, radiological, cardiac, neurologic examination	15.3/1,000 live births	Peng and Chuan, 1988
Medical records	10.2/1,000 births	Wu et al., 1995
Physical examination at birth Tests used to confirm clinically suspected cases: Radiological, hematological, serological, cardiac, neurological examination	5/1,000 births (major) 9/1,000 births (major and minor)	Masloman et al., 1991

TABLE A-1   continued

Country	Year	Population
India	1989–1992	Births, Jimper Hospital, Pondichery (live births 12,337 stillbirths 460) (n = 12,797)
India	1985–1986	Births, Mahatma Gandhi Institute of Medical Sciences and Civil Hospital, Wardha, (n = 3,014)
India	1981	Not specified
India	Not specified	Births, S. N. Medical college, Agra (n = 2,720)
India	Not specified	Births, Murnbai, Delhi and Baroda (n = 94,610)
India	Not specified	Births (n = 301,987)
Middle East and Eastern Europe		
United Arab Emirates	1998	Births (n = 4,861)
Hungary	1980–1994	Birth to 1 yr, five sources (n = not specified)

Method	Prevalence	Reference
Physical examination within 24 hours of birth Test used to confirm clinically suspected cases: Autopsy[a]	37/1,000 births (major and minor)	Bhat and Babu, 1998
Physical examination within 48 hours of birth Test used to confirm. clinically suspected cases: Radiological examination	20.6/1,000 births (major) 27.2/1,000 births (major and minor)	Chaturvedi and Banerjee, 1993
Indian census[b] data	25/1,000 births	Verma 1986
Physical examination within 48 hours of birth Test used to confirm clinically suspected cases: Further investigation	19.8/1,000 births	Kalra et al., 1984
Not specified	20.3/1,000 births	Verma et al., 1998
Meta-analysis	19.4/1,000 births	Verma et. al., 1990
Data source NCAR[c] Live births examined up to one year of life	30/1,000 births	Hosani and Czeizel, 2000
Data source[d]	Recorded 23/1,000 births (major) 46.3/1,000 births (major and minor) True 25.5/1,000 births (major) 65.3/1,000 births (major and minor)	Czeizel 1997

TABLE A-1 continued

Country	Year	Population
Hungary	1970–1980s	Not specified
Lebanon	1991–1993	Births (n = 3,865)
Latin America Brazil	1982–1985	Births, three maternity hospitals,^{f} Cubatao (n = 10,378)
Cuba	1982–1993	Pregnant women, 15–19 weeks' gestation, Havana (n = 356,380)
Developed Countries Japan	1948–1990	Births, St. Barnabas' Hospital, Osaka (live births 129,734, fetal deaths 2262) (n = 131,996)
United States	1968–1988	Births, Atlanta (n = 580,952)
	1989–1990	Births, Atlanta (n = 76,862)
Italy	1986–1989	Births (n = 448,195)
	1990	Births (n = 91,440)
South Korea	1993–1994	Infants <1 yr, Korean Federation of Medical Insurance (KFMI) 1993 (n = 601,376) 1994 (n = 601,459)

Method	Prevalence	Reference
Data source[e]	65/1,000	Czeizel et al., 1993
Physical examination within 24 hours of birth Tests used to confirm clinically suspected cases: Radiography, echography, brain scan, torch and chromosomal analysis	16.5/1,000 (major)	Bittar, 1998
ECLAMC[g] Wata physical examination at birth	10. 1/1,000 births (major) 15.3/1,000 births (major and minor)	Monteleone-Neto and Castilla 1994
Ultrasonography (USG) Maternal serum α-feto proteins (MS-AFP)	1982–1988 Raised MS-AFP 685 cases USG 686 cases	Rodríguez et al., 1997
Physical examination up to first week after birth	10.7/1,000 births	Imaizumi et al., 1991
MACDP[h] data	10/1,000 births 11/1,000 births	Khoury et al., 1993
IPIMC[i] data	8/1,000 births 8/1,000 births	Khoury et al., 1993
Data from KFMI	39.3/1,000 infants 1993 34.4/1,000 infants 1994	Jung et al., 1999

TABLE A-1   continued

Country	Year	Population
Turkey	1988–1995	Births, Gazi University, Ankara Referral Center Late termination of pregnancy included (*n* = 9,160)

[a]Stillbirths and neonatal deaths with parental consent.
[b]Data based on 1981 Indian census.
[c]National Congenital Abnormality Registry.
[d]Hungarian Congenital Abnormality Registry.
[e]Hungarian Congenital Abnormality Registry and medical records, all institutions.
[f]Oswaldo Cruz, Ana Costa and De Cubatao.
[g]Latin American Collaborative Study of Congenital Malformations.
[h]Metropolitan Atlanta Congenital Defects Program.
[i]Italian Multi-Centric Register of Congenital Malformations.

Method	Prevalence	Reference
Physical examination at birth	11.1/1,000 births	Himmetoglu et al., 1996

TABLE A-2 Studies on the Prevalence of Down Syndrome

Country	Year	Population
Africa		
South Africa	1974–1993	Births[a], Cape Town
	1974	(n = 20,358)
	1993	(n = 31,446)
South Africa	1980–1984	Live births,[d] white population, Pretoria (n = 384,197) Live births (n = 4,939,640)
South Africa	1989–1992	Live births, Mankweng Hospital, Sovenga, Northern Transvaal (n = 7,617)
Libya	1985	Live births, Jamahirya Maternity Hospital, Benghazi (n = 16,000)
Nigeria	1972–1980	Live births, Ibadan (n = 3,000)
Asia		
Malaysia	1986–1987	Live births, Maternity Hospital, Kuala Lumpur (n = 34,522)
Malaysia	1986–1987	Live births, Maternity Hospital, Kuala Lumpur (n = 34,495)

Method	Prevalence	Reference

Data source[b]
Test used to confirm
clinically suspected
cases:
  Chromosomal
  analysis[c]
	1.5/1,000 births
	
	1.4/1,000 births
	
	1.2/1,000 births
		Molteno et
		al., 1997

Prenatal diagnosis, source[e]	0.5/1,000 live births	Op't Hof et al., 1991
Pooled data, six large studies[f]	1.3/1,000 live births	
Physical examination within 24 hours of birth	2.1/1,000 live births	Venter et al., 1995

Physical examination
Test used to confirm
clinically suspected
cases:
  Chromosome
  analysis (cultures
  and G-banding of
  karyotype)
	1.9/1,000 live
	births
		Verma et
		al., 1990

Hospital records[g]	1.2/1,000 live births	Adeyokunnu, 1982

Physical examination
Test used to confirm
clinically suspected
cases:
  Chromosomal
  analysis
	1/1,000 live births
	
	Malay
	1/1,000 live births
	Chinese
	1/1,000 live births
	Indians
	1.2/1,000 live births
		Hoe et al.,
		1989

Physical examination
Test used to confirm
clinically suspected
cases:
  Chromosomal
  analysis
	1/1,000 live births	Boo et al., 1989

TABLE A-2 continued

Country	Year	Population
Indonesia	1983–1987	Births, Gunung Wenang Hospital Manado, Jakarta ($n = 13,354$)
Pakistan	1984	Births ($n = 1,134$)
India	1985–1986	Births, Mahatma Gandhi Institute of Medical Sciences, Wardha Maharashtra ($n = 3,014$)
India	1976–1978	Live births, Niloufer hospital, Hyderabad ($n = 9,389$)
India	Not specified	Births, multicentric study, Mumbai, Delhi, Baroda ($n = 94,610$)
India	Not specified	Births, Delhi, Patna, Bombay, Madras, Trivandrum, Ajmer, ($n = 75,103$)
Middle East Saudi Arabia	1982–1991	Live births to Saudi mothers, King Khalid university hospital Riyadh ($n = 23,261$) Live births to non-Saudi mothers ($n = 4,920$)

Method	Prevalence	Reference
Physical examination at birth Tests used to confirm clinically suspected cases: Radiological, hematological, serological, cardiac, neurological examination	0.1/1,000 births	Masloman et al., 1991
Physical examination within first week of life	4.4/1,000 births	Jalil et al., 1993
Physical examination within 48 hours of birth	0.7/1,000 births	Chaturvedi and Banerjee, 1989
Hospital records Physical examination at birth Test used to confirm clinically suspected cases: Cytogenetic analysis	1.2/1,000 live births	Isaac et al., 1985
Physical examination at birth Test used to confirm clinically suspected cases: Cytogenetic analysis	0.9/1,000 births	Verma et al., 1998
Meta-analysis Physical examination at birth cytogenetic analysis when possible	1.1/1,000 births	Verma et al., 1988
Hospital records[h] Physical examination at birth Test used to confirm clinically suspected cases: Cytogenetic analysis	1.8/1,000 Saudi live births 1.8/1,000 non-Saudi live births Overall 1.8/1,000 live births	Niazi et al., 1995

TABLE A-2 continued

Country	Year	Population
Latin America		
Argentina	1967–1995	Births in 53 hospitals (n = 1,668,733)
Brazil	1982–1986	Births, three participating hospitals, Cubatao, (n = 10,378)
Developed Countries		
Kuwait	1986	Live births, 2 district hospitals Jahra[j] (n = 300,000) Births, Farwania[k] (n = 400,000)
Israel	1984	Live births (n = 86,833)
	1980	Live births (n = 85,575)
Israel	1979	Live births to mothers 35 years or older (n = 69,896)
	1992	Live births (n = 78,442)

[a]Includes live births, stillbirths, and terminated pregnancies.
[b]The Department of Human Genetics of the University of Cape Town, Cape Mental Health Society Register, and Down Syndrome Association records.
[c]All but three cases confirmed.
[d]Live births among whites, with 1-year interval of maternal age obtained from State Central Statistical Services.
[e]Central cytogenetic database, Genetic Services Division, South Africa.
[f]New York, Ohio, British Columbia, Massachusetts, Sweden, and Clanmorgan.
[g]University College Hospital, Ibadan.
[h]Neonatal unit registries, pediatric department, cytogenetic laboratory, and computer-based medical records.
[i]Latin American Collaborative Study of Congenital Malformations.
[j]80 percent Bedouin population.
[k]15 percent Bedouin population.
[l]Maternal and Child Health Department of the Ministry of Health.
[m]National Program for Detection and Prevention of Birth Defects of the Israel Ministry of Health.

Method	Prevalence	Reference
ECLAMC[i] data	Lowland 1.6/1,000 births	Castilla et al., 1999
	Highland 1.4/1,000 births	
ECLAMC data Physical examination	1.2/1,000 births	Monteleone-Neto and Castilla, 1994
Community genetic survey	3.6/1,000 live births	Al-Awadi et al., 1990
	1.5/1,000 births	
Data source[l]	1/1,000 live births	Kalir, 1985
	0.9/1,000 live births	
Data source[m]	1/1,000 live births	Shohat et al., 1995
	0.5/1,000 live births	

TABLE A-3   Studies on the Prevalence of Thalassemia

Country	Year	Population
Asia		
Thailand	1997–1998	Pregnant women, Antenatal Clinic, Ramathibodi Hospital (n = 8,763) Couples (n = 1,840)
China	1986–1987	Chinese women, antenatal clinic, health centers and government hospital, Macau (n = 3,815) Cord blood sample (n = 1,091)
India	1999	Children, six Ashram schools, aged 6–15 yr, . Orrisa (n = 465)
Middle East and Eastern Europe		
Jordan	1989	Alternate outpatients, aged 2–80 yr, Princess Basma teaching hospital, Irbid (n = 1,000)
Jordan	1989	Children randomly selected, aged 6–10 yr (n = 456)
Jordan	Not specified	Volunteers, Northern Jordan (3 regions) (n = 2,290) Live births (n = 568)
Turkey	1995–1999	Couples, marriage registry office, and Regional Health Administration, Denizili (province) (n = 9,902)

Method	Prevalence	Reference
MCV^a < 80 femtoliters (fL), high performance liquid chromatography	Couples at risk[b] 4%	Jaovisidha et al., 2000
MCH^c < 27 picograms (pg), Hb^d electrophoresis-cellulose acetate	β-Thalassemia carriers 3.4%	Tamagnini et al., 1988
Isoelectric focusing (IEF) — polyacylamide gel and Hb^d Bart's	α-Thalassemia carriers 6.2%	
Hb^d electrophoresis-cellulose acetate	β-Thalassemia carriers 3.0%	Balgir et al., 1999
MCV^a < 75 fL, Hb^d electrophoresis-cellulose acetate, microchromatography	α-Thalassemia carriers 3.5% β-Thalassernia minor 3.1 %	Bashir et al., 1992
Complete blood count MCV^a < 75 fL, Hb^d electrophoresis-cellulose acetate and paragon gels (Beckman), HbA2 level— microcolumn chromatography	β-Thalassemia minor 3.3% β-Thalassemia carrier 3.5%	Bashir et al., 1991
Hb^d electrophoresis	β-Thalassernia 5.93%	Sunna et al., 1996
MCV^a < 80 fL, Hb^d electrophoresis-cellulose acetate, HbA2 level	β-Thalassemia carriers 2.6%	Keskin et al., 2000

TABLE A-3   continued

Country	Year	Population
Developed Countries		
Hong Kong	1988–1997	Pregnant women, < 18 weeks' gestation, Kwong Wah Hospital (n = 25,834)
Sardinia	Not specified	Males, females, married couples, and pregnant women (n = 167,000)
Cyprus	1984	Males and females, Turkish Cypriots, North Cyprus (n = 1365)
Cyprus	1974–1979	Males and females, Cyprus (n = 18,344)

[a]MCV = Mean corpuscular volume.
[b]Couples at risk of having a child with homozygous β-thalassemia or β-thalassemia-HbE disease.
[c]Mean corpuscular hemoglobin.
[d]Hb = hemoglobin; RBC = red blood cell.
[e]Percentage is higher because, prior to 1976, relatives of patients were specifically sought for screening.

Method	Prevalence	Reference
MCV[a] <75 fL, HbA2 level >3.5%	α-Thalassemia carriers 4.3%	Sin et al., 2000
	β-Thalassemia carriers 2.8% α-, β- Thalassemia carriers 0.1%	
RBC[d] indices, Hb[d] electrophoresis, HbA2 level	β-Thalassemia carriers 30,000 Couples at risk 1,544	Cao et al., 1991
Hb[d] electrophoresis- cellulose acetate	β-Thalassemia carriers 14.4%	Cin at al., 1984
Hematological indices, blood film examination, cellulose acetate electrophoresis, osmotic fragility, HbF measurement, globin chain separation	β-Thalassemia carriers 19.4%[e]	Angastiniotis and Hadjiminas, 1981

TABLE A-4 Studies on the Prevalence of Sickle Cell Disease

Country	Year	Population
Africa		
Nigeria	Not specified	Randomly selected males and females, aged >15 yr, 30 states (n = 16,000)
Sierra Leone	1990–1993	Routine checkups and patients with anemia symptoms, Ramsy Medical Laboratories (n = 3,524)
Latin America		
Brazil	1980	Mixed parentage (n = 8,830)
		Whites (n = 17,584)
		Blacks (n = 7,747)
Cuba	1983	Couples (n = 19,686)
Cuba	1989	Pregnant women nationwide (n = 806,935)
Asia		
Pakistan	Over 2 yr not specified	All inpatients, Medical Unit, Jinnah Postgraduate Medical Center, Karachi (n = 2,080)
India	1981–1985	Randomly selected outpatients, tribal clinics, Tamil Nadu (n = 1,377)
India	1986	Hospitalized patients in Orissa (n = 9,822)
	Not specified	Males and females randomly selected, regional population, Orissa (n = 1,000)

Method	Prevalence	Reference
Nigerian national survey	S gene 25.3% HbAS 23% HbAC 1.8% HbSS 0.3% HbSC 0.2%	Angastiniotis et al., 1995
Sickling test Hb electrophoresis	HbS 22% HbAS 7.5% HbSS & HbSC 2.2%	Wurie et al., 1996
Brazilian census^a data	HbAS 4.7% HbSS 0.2% Others 1.7% HbAS 0.9% HbSS 0.1% Others 0.7% HbAS 6.2% HbSS 0.3% Others 1.6%	Salzano, 1985
Nationwide screening	Both partners carriers 6.4%	Granda et al., 1994
Nationwide prenatal diagnosis	SC anemia carriers 3.7% HbAS 3% HbAC 0.65% HbSS 0.02% HbSC 0.02% Others 0.04%	Granda et al., 1994
Sickling test Hb electrophoresis	Sickle cell disease 3.5% (HbS/D-Punjab 37.5% HbS/thalassemia 62.5%)	Kazmi and Rab, 1990
Solubility test Hb electrophoresis	HbAS (30–37.8%) HbSS (1.2–1.9%)	Ramasamy et al., 1994
Sickling test Hb electrophoresis	S gene in hospitalized patients 11.1 % Incidence of S gene in the surveyed population 15.1%	Kar, 1991

TABLE A-4   continued

Country	Year	Population
India	1995–1996	All pediatric inpatients, Kusturba Hospital, Maharashtra (*n* = 1,753)
India	Not specified	Randomly selected males and females (*n* = 2,570) Kerala (973) Madhya Pradesh (696) Orissa (901)
India	1991	Children, six Ashram Schools, aged 6–15 yr, Orrisa (*n* = 465)
India	Over 10 yr	Tribal population, Maharashtra (*n* = 7.4 million)
Middle East		
Saudi Arabia	Not specified 1982–1994	Males, Saudi Arabia (*n* = 840)
Saudi Arabia		Males and females, Ministry of Health hospitals and primary health care centers and volunteers, King Saud University (*n* = 30,055)
Jordan	1989	Children randomly selected, aged 6–10 yr (*n* = 456)
Jordan	1989	Alternate out-patients, aged 2–80 yr, Princess Basma Teaching Hospital, Irbid (*n* = 1,000)
Jordan	Not specified	Volunteers, Northern Jordan (3 regions) (*n* = 2,290) Live births (*n* = 568)
Jordan	Not specified	Live births, Irbid (*n* = 181) Males 90 Females 91

*a*1980 Brazilian census; ethnic distribution according to the 1950 census.

Method	Prevalence	Reference
Sickling test Hb electrophoresis	Sickle cell disease 5.7% HbAS 3.5% HbSS 2.2%	Kamble and Chaturvedi, 2000
Sickling test Hb electrophoresis	HbAS (9.93–32.38%) HbSS (0.68–16.25)	Kaur et al., 1997
Physical examination Sickling test Hb electrophoresis	HbAS 0.6%	Balgir et al., 1999
Solubility test Hb electrophoresis	HbAS 10% HbSS 0.5%	Kate, 2000
Sickling test Hb electrophoresis	HbS 5.7%	Ganeshaguru, et al., 1987
Hb electrophoresis	HbAS 7.4% HbSS 1.1%	El-Hazmi et al., 1996
Sickling test Hb elcetrophoresis- cellulose acetate and paragon gels (Beckman)	HbAS 0.44%	Bashir et al., 1991
Solubility test Hb electrophoresis	HbAS 1% Estimated HbSS at birth 0.25%	Bashir et al., 1992
Hb electrophoresis	HbS 4.5% HbSS 1.3%, HbSA 3.3% HbAS 3.2%	Sunna et al., 1996
Hb electrophoresis	HbS 5% Male 6% Female 4%	Talafih et al., 1996

TABLE A-5   Studies on the Prevalence of Glucose-6-Phosphate
Dehydrogenase Deficiency

Country	Year	Population
Africa		
Libya	1984	Births, Jamahiriya Maternity Hospital, Benghazi (n = 120)
		Males and females[a] (n = 320)
Asia		
Malaysia	1983–1984	Births, Malacca (n = 12,579)
Thailand	1996–1998	Births, Rajavithi Hospital, Bangkok (n = 24,714)
Taiwan	1987–1997[c]	Births, 1,143 delivery units, Taipei (n = 2,971,192)
Pakistan	1989	Male school children[d], aged 5–14 yr
		Pakistani Pathans (n = 100) Afghan refugees Pathan (n = 14) Turkoman (n = 92) Uzbek (n = 33) Tajik (n = 35)
India	Not specified	Births, Christian Medical College, Ludhiana (n = 1,000)
India	1994	Births, 13 hospitals, Bangalore, Karnataka (n = 5,140)

Method	Prevalence	Reference
Dichlorophenol indophenol fluorescent spot test G6PD[b] erythrocyte activity Hemograms Reticulocyte count	Male population 2.8%	Mir et al., 1985
Fluorescent spot test	Total 2.3% Chinese 3.2%, Malays 2.3%, Indians 1.3%	Singh, 1986
Fluorescent spot test	Total 5.1% Males 9.1% Females 1.7%	Ratrisawadi et al., 1999
Quantitative fluorescent spot test Test used to confirm clinically suspected cases: Semiquantitative fluorometric test	Total 2.1% Male 3.1% Females 0.9%	Chiang et al., 1999
Survey Test used to confirm clinically suspected cases: Quantitative visual colorimetric determination	Pakistani Pathans 7% Afghan Pathan Refugees 15.8% Turkoman 2.2% Uzbek 9.1% Tajik 2.9%	Bouma et al., 1995
Modified fluorescent spot test QMRT[e] Hemoglobin count, reticulocyte count, peripheral blood smear[f]	Total 3.9% Males 5% Females 2.8%	Verma et al., 1990
Electrophoresis	7.8%	Ramadevi et al., 1994

TABLE A-5 continued

Country	Year	Population
India	1999	Children, six Ashram schools, age 6–15 yr Orissa ($n = 465$)
Middle East and Eastern Europe		
Turkey	1986–1988	Males and females, randomly selected, 375 families, Antalya city and adjacent village ($n = 1,521$)
North Cyprus	1984	Males and females, healthy Turkish Cypriots ($n = 250$)
Iraq	1972	Males[h], Republic Hospital, Baghdad ($n = 563$)
Iraq	1972	Live births, two maternity Hospitals, Baghdad ($n = 889$)
Iraq	1994	Births, randomly selected, Basrah Maternity and Al-Tahreer Hospital, Basrah ($n = 1,226$) Healthy university students, aged 20–35, Basrah ($n = 498$)
Developed Countries		
Singapore	Over 7 years	Births, National University Hospital ($n = 22,830$)

Method	Prevalence	Reference
Physical examination Hb electrophoresis	9.2%	Balgir et al., 1999
Beutler's fluorescent spot test Modified Zinkham method G6PD[b] chemical characterization[g]	Males 7.4% Females 1.8%	Aksu et al., 1990
Not specified	12.4%	Cin et al., 1984
Beutler's and Fairbanks fluorescent spot test	Males 8.4%	Amin-Zaki et al., 1972
Beutler's and Fairbanks fluorescent spot test	Live births 8.9%	Amin-Zaki et al., 1972
Modified Beutler method G6PD[b] activity[i] Hexokinase activity Pyruvate kinase activity	Males 7.9% births Females 9.7% births	Al-Naama et al., 1994
	Male students 9.2%, Females students 11.8%	
Enzyme activity: Wong's in-house modified Bernstein's technique Quantitative estimation of enzyme activity: based on Beutler assay	Total 1.6% Males 3.2% Females 0.1% Variation among males Chinese 3.9%, Malays 2.9%, Indians 0.7%	Joseph et al., 1999

TABLE A-5 continued

Country	Year	Population
Hong Kong	1995	Births, Chinese origin, University Maternity Hospital (*n* = 1,228)
Greece	1977–1989	Births, 174 national and private maternity units (*n* = 1,286,000)
Greece	Not specified	Adult blood samples, Blood Donation Department, Speliopouleion General Hospital, Athens (*n* = 2,150) Births, maternity hospital, Greater Athens (*n* = 2,400)

*a*Includes 120 mothers and 200 healthy males (medical students, staff and blood donors).
*b*G6PD = Glucose-6-phosphate dehydrogenase.
*c*Nationwide screening using heel blood sample from infants at 1143 delivery units in Taiwan in 1997. Coverage rate of neonatal screening 99%.
*d*Refugees of Yakka, Ghund, Mohmand agency, Khorasan and Barakai.
*e*Quantitative methemoglobin reduction test used to confirm all nonfluorescent and partially fluorescent cases.
*f*Cases were checked for hemolysis.
*g*World Health Organization (WHO) standardized procedure for study of G6PD—1976.
*h*Medical students, blood donors, and hospitalized patients.
*i*Measured according to the World Health Organization (WHO) method.
*j*Sansone method, classic Beutler method used occasionally.

Method	Prevalence	Reference
Modified fluorescent spot test G6PD[b] enzyme level	Males 4.5% Females 0.4%	Fok et al., 1985
Fluorescent spot test Spectrophotometric method Sansone method classic Beutler method[i]	Total 3.14% Males 4.5% Females 1.8%	Missiou-Tsagaraki, 1991
Beutler assay using quantase MMR500 G6PD[b] screening kit	Adults 5.5%	Reclos et al., 2000
	Births 3.1%	

TABLE A-6   Studies on the Prevalence of Oculocutaneous Albinism

Country	Year	Population
Africa		
South Africa	1989–1992	Live births[a], Mankweng Hospital, Northern Transvaal (*n* = 7,617)
South Africa	1986–1989	Live births, Kalafong Hospital, Pretoria (*n* = 17,351)
South Africa	1970	Black population, Soweto, Johannesburg[c] (*n* = 803,511)
Cameroon	1972–1987	Population, 1976 national census (*n* = 7,663,246) Bamilekes, Cameroon (*n* = 1,500,000)
Zimbabwe	Not specified	Community population, Tonga (*n* = 11,000)
Zimbabwe	Not specified	Children, aged 6–23 yr, 1747 schools outside Harare (*n* = 1.3 million)
Zimbabwe	1994	Children, aged 12–22 yr, 69 schools, Harare (*n* = 87,817)
Nigeria	1950	Schoolchildren, aged 4–20 yr, Lagos and outlying districts (*n* = 14,292)
Asia		
Indonesia	1983–1987	Births, Gunung Wenang Hospital, Manado, Jakarta (*n* = 13,354)

Method	Prevalence	Reference
Physical examination within 24 hours of birth[b]	1/1,523 live births	Venter et al., 1995
Physical examination within 24 hours of birth	0.23/1,000 live births	Delport et al., 1995
Survey, 120 schools, 6 health clinics, St. John's Eye Hospital, Baragwanath Hospital, welfare organizations, municipal social workers, and families with albinism	Albinism 1/3,900 Carrier rate 1/32 (Southern Sotho 1/2,254, Xhosa 1/4,700, Pedi 1/9,700, Shangaan people 1/28,614)	Kromberg and Jenkins, 1982
Physical examination interview and genetic marker testing	1/35,000 (1978) 1/28,000 (1987) 1/11,900 (1978) 1/7,900 (1987)	Aquaron, 1990
Postal survey follow-up. PCR[d] analysis	1/1,000	Lund et al., 1997
Postal survey[e]	1/4,728	Lund, 1996
Postal survey[f]	1/2,661	Kagore and Lund, 1995
Postal survey	1/2,858	Barnicot, 1952
Medical records[g]	1/4,451	Masloman et al., 1991

TABLE A-6 continued

Country	Year	Population
Latin America		
Cuba		Cuna Indian population
	1925	(n = 20,100)
	1940	(n = 20,831)
	1950	(n = 22,822)
	1962	(n = 23,743)
	1970	(n = 24,800)

[a]Neonatal deaths included.
[b]Observation, palpation, and measurement of newbom according to genetic service division, Department of National Health and Population Development.
[c]National Census, 1970.
[d]PCR = polymerase chain reaction.
[e]Fifty cases confirmed by physical examination.
[f]Cases confirmed by physical examination.
[g]Cases identified by physical examination at birth confirmed with special procedures when required.
[h]Studies conducted in the same town.

Method	Prevalence	Reference
Physical examination[b]		Harris and Prieto, 1925
	69/10,000	Stout, 1942
	47/10,000	Keeler, 1950
	67/10,000	Keeler and Prieto,
	61/10,000	1964
	63/10,000	Keeler, 1970

TABLE A-7   Studies on the Prevalence of Cystic Fibrosis

Country	Year	Population
Africa		
Africa	Not specified	African blacks, southern, central, and western Africa (n = 1,360)
Middle East and Eastern Europe		
Bahrain	1978–1995	Not specified
Turkey	Not specified	Births, maternity clinic, Istanbul (n = 6,061)
Jordan	1990–1999	Live births, Rahman Teaching Hospital, Irbid and Islamic Hospital, Amman (n = 1,260,000)
Jordan	Not specified	Live births, 10 hospitals, Amman, Zarqa, Irbid, Jarash (n = 7,682)
Developed Countries		
Israel	1981–1987	Live births, Israel (n = 516,908) Europe–America, Jews (n = 207,111) Asia-Africa, Jews (n = 309,797)

aPCR = polymerase chain reaction.
bMinistry of Health database and Department of Pediatrics medical records.
cChloride electrode and neutron activation analysis.
dUsing pilocarpine electophoresis.
eCases confirmed by sweat test.
fDNA analysis with PCR conducted in 50 cases.

Method	Prevalence	Reference
DNA analysis, PCR assay[a]	1/128 carriers	Padoa et al., 1999
Medical records [b]	1/5,800 Bahraini live births 1/33,333 population	Al-Mahroos, 1998
Sweat chloride test[c]	1/3,000 births	Gurson et al., 1973
Sweat test [d]	1/8,129 live births	Rawashdeh and Manal, 2000
Boehringer Mannheim (BM) meconium test[e]	1/2,560 live births	Nazer, 1992
Physical examination Sweat chloride test[f]	1/5,221 live births 1/3,288 live births	Kerem et al., 1995
	1/9,388 live births Ashkenazi 1/3,300 Libya 1/2,700 Georgia 1/2,700 Greece/Bulgaria 1/2,400 Yemen 1/8,800 Morocco 1/15,000 Iraq 1/32,000 Iran 1/39,000	

TABLE A-8   Studies on the Prevalence of Phenylketonuria

Country	Year	Population
Africa		
South Africa	1979–1986	Births, whites, Pretoria ($n = 59,600$)
Asia		
China	1982–1985	Births, 11 provinces and cities [b] ($n = 198,320$)
China	1992–1997	Births, 8 cities[e] (n 1,107,212)
Middle East and Eastern Europe		
Czech Republic	1974–1975	Births, screening center, Prague ($n = 132,392$)
Poland	1974–1975	Births, screening center, Warsaw ($n = 894,891$)
Iran	1982	Births, hospitals, Tehran ($n = 8,633$)
Estonia	1993–1995	Births, maternity hospitals[b] ($n = 36,074$)
	1980–1992	Not specified

Method	Prevalence	Reference
Thin-layer chromatography[a]	1/20,000 births	Hitzeroth et al., 1995
Guthrie test[c]	Beijing City 1/15,200 births Tiajnin and Hebei 1/7,600 births[d] Shanghai and East China 1/45,300 births[d] Northeast China 1/12,800 births Western China 0/25,800 births[d]	Liu and Zuo, 1986
Guthrie test Flurometric enzyme immunoassay[f]	Total 1/14,767 births Shanghai 1/17,580 births Beijing 1/11,379 births Guangzhou 1/37,036 births Tianjin 1/5,124 births Nanjing 1/12,617 births Shenyang 1/36,251 births Jinan 0/38,732 births Chengdu 1/38,933 births	Fan et al., 1999
Guthrie test	1/6,618 births	Collaborative study, 1975
Guthrie test	1/7,782 births	Collaborative study, 1975
Guthrie test[g]	1/8,000 births	Farhud and Kabiri, 1982
Modified fluorometric method	1/6,010 births	Ounap et al., 1998
Medical records[i]	1/8,090 births	

TABLE A-8   continued

Country	Year	Population
Turkey	Not specified	Births, maternity hospital, metropolitan districts[j] (n = 170,466)
Latvia		Births (n = 500,000+)

[a]Screening program conducted by National Health and Population Development.
[b]Beijing, Tianjin, Shanghai, Hebei, Shandong, Zhejiang, Leioning, Jilin, Heilongjiang, Sichuan, Shanxi.
[c]Guthrie's bacterial inhibition assay.
[d]Including one case of hyperphenylalaninemia.
[e]Shanghai, Beijing, Guangzhou, Tianjin, Nanjing, Shenyang, Jinan, Chengdu.
[f]Used by one of the laboratories to diagnose phenylketonuria.
[g]Examined within 4–6 days of birth.
[h]Data from health authorities of Estonia.
[i]All Estonia regional children's outpatient department and genetic counseling records of Tallinn outpatient clinic.
[j]Ankara, Istanbul, Izmir, Samsun, Trabzon, and Diyarbakir.

Method	Prevalence	Reference
Guthrie test	1/4,370 births	Ozalp et al., 1990
Fluorometric method	1/8,700 births	Lugovska et al., 1999

Tests used to
confirm clinically
suspected cases:
 Amino acid
 analysis
 DNA analysis

TABLE A-9 Studies on the Prevalence of Neural Tube Defects (NTDs) and Hydrocephalus[a]

Country	Year	Population	Method
Africa			
South Africa	1976–1977	Births (n = 29,633)	Data from pediatric ward and mortuary records
South Africa	1989–1992	Births, Mankweng Hospital (n = 7,617)	Physical examination within 24 hours of birth
South Africa	1973–1992	Births, hospitals, Capetown (n = 516,252)	Hospital records
South Africa	1986–1989	Live births, Kalafong Hospital, Pretoria (n = 17,351)	Physical examination within 24 hours of birth
Tunisia	1983–1984	Births, Wassila Bourgiba Hospital, Tunis (n = 10,000)	Physical examination within 24 hours of birth
Zimbabwe	1984	Births, Harare Maternity Hospital and clinics, Greater Harare (n = 18,033) Neonatal admissions, Harare (n = 2,154)	Medical records

Prevalence	Type of NTD	Reference
1.2/1,000 births	Spina bifida and anencephaly	Kromberg and Jenkins, 1982
1.3/1,000 births	Hydrocephalus	
3.5/1,000 births	NTDs	Venter et al., 1995
1.7/1,000 births	Anencephaly	
1.6/1,000 births	Spina bifida	
0.3/1,000 births	Encephalocele	
0.5/1,000 births	Hydrocephalus	
Whites 2.6/1,000 births Blacks 0.9/1,000 births Mixed parentage 1/1,000 births	NTDs	Buccimazza et al., 1994
0.2/1,000 live births	Anencephaly	Delport et al., 1995
0.5/1,000 live births	Spina bifida	
0.3/1,000 live births	Spina bifida with hydrocephalus	
0.1/1,000 live births	Encephalocele	
0.6/1,000 live births	Hydrocephalus	
0.6/1,000 births	Anencephaly	Khrouf et al., 1986
0.9/1,000 births	Hydrocephalus	
1.3/1,000 births	Spina bifida	
0.2/1,000 births	Spina bifida	Shija and Kingo, 1985

TABLE A-9 continued

Country	Year	Population	Method
Nigeria	1987–1990	Births,[b] Jos University Teaching Hospital, Jos (n = 5,977)	Physical examination within 24 hours of birth
Tanzania	1985	Dar es Salaam	Not specified
Asia			
China	1980–1987	Births, 42 hospitals, South and North China	Not specified
China	1988–1991	Births, National Center for Birth Defects Monitoring (n = 2,750,588)	Hospital records
China	1986–1990	Births, rural area (n = 167,274)	Not specified
China	1986–1987	Births (live and stillbirths), >28 weeks of gestation, 945 hospitals, 29 provinces (n = 1,243,284)	Physical examination at birth Data source[c]
Indonesia	1983–1987	Births, Gunung Wenang Hospital, Manado Jakarta (n = 13,354)	Hospital records
Pakistan	1984	Births (n = 1,134)	Physical examination within first week of life

Prevalence	Type of NTD	Reference
7/1,000 births	NTDs	Airede, 1992
0.3/1,000 births	Spina bifida	Shija and Kingo, 1985
South China 1.6/1,000 births	NTDs	Melnick and Marazita, 1998
North China 7.3/1,000 births		
2.5/1,000 births 1.5/1,000 births 0.8/1,000 births 0.4/1,000 births	NTDs Anencephaly Spina bifida Encephalocele	Wu et al., 1995
2/1,000 births	Neural system birth defects	Hu et al., 1996 (in Chinese)
0.9/1,000 births 0.4/1,000 births 0.9/1,000 births	Anencephaly Spina bifida Hydrocephalus	
1.5/1,000 births 0.8/1,000 births 0.4/1,000 births 2.7/1,000 births 0.9/1,000 births	Anencephaly Spina bifida Encephalocele NTDs Hydrocephalus	Xiao et al., 1990
0.3/1,000 births 0.2/1,000 births	Anencephaly Hydrocephalus	Masloman et al., 1991
7.9/1,000 births	NTDs	Jalil et al., 1993

TABLE A-9   continued

Country	Year	Population	Method
India	1989–1992	Births, Jimper Hospital, Pondicherry (live births 12,337 stillbirths 460) (n = 12,797)	Physical examination within 24 hours of birth Autopsy[d]
India	1984	Births, J.J-M. Medical College, Karnataka (n = 2,000)	Physical examination at birth
India	1984	Births, 3 hospitals, Karnataka (n = 3,500)	Physical examination within 24 hours of birth Autopsy
India	Not specified	Births, Obstetrics Department, S.N. Medical College, Agra (n = 2,720)	Physical examination within 48 hours of birth
India	Not specified	Live and stillbirths, North India (n = 58,445) Live births, Bombay (n = 153,811) Live and stillbirths, Madras (n = 23,315) Live and stillbirths, Calcutta (n = 136,246) Live and stillbirths, Pondicherry (n = 14,482)	Data from published and unpublished sources, different hospitals in India

Prevalence	Type of NTD	Reference
0.5/1,000 births	Anencephaly	Bhat and Babu, 1998
0.2/1,000 births	Spina bifida	
0.7/1,000 births	Meningomyelocele	
0.2/1,000 births	Encephalocele	
1.6/1,000 births	Hydrocephalus	
11/1,000 births	NTDs	Kulkarni et al., 1998
11.4/1,000 births	NTDs	Kulkarni et al., 1989
5.1/1,000 births	Anencephaly	
3.1/1,000 births	Meningomyelocele	
0.8/1,000 births	Encephalocele	
2.6/1,000 births	Anencephaly	Kalra et al., 1984
2.2/1,000 births	Spina bifida	
1.5/1,000 births	Encephalocele	
2.2/1,000 births	Hydrocephalus	
4.8/1,000 births	Anencephaly	Verma, 1978
2.3/1,000 births	Spina bifida	
7.1/1,000 births	Anencephaly + spina bifida	
1.3/1,000 births	Anencephaly	
0.9/1,000 births	Spina bifida	
2.2/1,000 births	Anencephaly + spina bifida	
1.3/1,000 births	Anencephaly	
1.0/1,000 births	Spina bifida	
2.3/1,000 births	Anencephaly + spina bifida	
0.6/1,000 births	Anencephaly	
0.2/1,000 births	Spina bifida	
0.8/1,000 births	Anencephaly + spina bifida	
0.9/1,000 births	Anencephaly	
1/1,000 births	Spina bifida	
1.9/1,000 births	Anencephaly + spina bifida	

TABLE A-9   continued

Country	Year	Population	Method
India	1982–1991	Births, 4 hospitals[e] Lucknow (n = 129,676)	Hospital records
India	1985–1986	Births, Mahatma Gandhi Institute of Medical Sciences and Civil Hospital, Wardha, (n = 3,014)	Physical examination within 48 hours of birth Test used to confirm clinically suspected cases: Radiological examination
Middle East Northern Jordan	1991–1993	Live births, Irbid (n = 86,812)	Hospital records[f]
Saudi Arabia	1996–1997	Live births, Maternity and Children's Hospital and Ohud Hospital, Al-Madinah Al-Munawarah (n = 16,550)	Physical examination within 28 days of life
Latin America Brazil	1982–1986	Births, 3 participating Hospitals (n = 10,378)	ECLAMC[g] data
Developed Countries United States	1968–1988	Births, Atlanta (n = 580,952)	MACDP[h] data
United Kingdom	Not specified	Liverpool	Not specified

Prevalence	Type of NTD	Reference
3.9/1,000 births	NTD	Sharma et al., 1994
	Anencephaly and spina bifida	
1.3/1,000 births	Anencephaly	Chaturvedi and
1.3/1,000 births	Hydrocephalus	Banerjee, 1989
0.3/1,000 births	Meningocele	
0.7/1,000 births	Meningomyelocele	
0.3/1,000 births	Meningoencephalocele	
1.6/1,000 live births	NTDs	Daoud et al., 1997
0.4/1,000 live births	Anencephaly	
1.0/1,000 live births	Spina bifida	
0.3/1,000 live births	Encephalocele	
1.6/1,000 live births	Hydrocephalus	Murshid et al., 2000
0.5/1,000 births	Anencephaly	Monteleone-
0.3/1,000 births	Spina bifida	Neto and Castilla,
0.2/1,000 births	Hydrocephalus	1994
0.5/1,000 births	Anencephaly	Khoury et al., 1993
0.8/1,000 births	Spina bifida	
0.2/1,000 births	Encephalocele	
0.9/1,000 births	Hydrocephalus	
2.6/1,000 births	Anencephaly	Shija and Kingo, 1985
3.1/1,000 births	Spina bifida	

TABLE A-9 continued

Country	Year	Population	Method
Italy	1986–1989	Births (n = 448,195)	IPIMC[i] data
Israel	1980–1984	Births in 1984 (n = 86,833)	Data source[j]
Argentina	1967–1995	Births, 53 hospitals (n = 1,668,733)	ECLAMC data
South Korea	1993–1994	Infants <1 yr, Korean Federation of Medical Insurance	Data from KFMI[k]
	1993	(n = 601,376)	
	1994	(n = 601,459)	
World			
World	Not specified	Not specified	Not specified

[a]Hydrocephalus is excessive accumulation of cerebrospinal fluid, which is frequently associated with neural tube defects.
[b]Includes stillbirths and neonatal births.
[c]Chinese Birth Defects Monitoring Program.
[d]Includes stillbirths and neonatal deaths with parental consent.
[e]Queen Mary's, Mahila Aspatal, Fatima, Vivekanand Hospital.

Prevalence	Type of NTD	Reference
0.1/1,000 births	Anencephaly	Khoury et al., 1993
0.4/1,000 births	Spina bifida	
0.1/1,000 births	Encephalocele	
0.4/1,000 births	Hydrocephalus	
0.1/1,000 births	Anencephalus	Kalir, 1985
0.4/1,000 births	Spina bifida	
0.1/1,000 births	Spina bifida with hydrocephalus	
0.1/1,000 births	Hydrocephalus	
0.05/1,000 births	Encephalocele	
Lowland 0.5/1,000 births Highland 0.2/1,000 births	Anencephaly	Castilla et al., 1999
0.6/1,000 (LL) 0.3/1,000 (HL)	Spina bifida	
0.4/1,000 (LL) 0.1/1,000 (HL)	Hydrocephalus	
0.3–0.4/1,000	Anencephaly	Jung et al., 1999
0.30–0.27/1,000	Spina bifida	
0.11–0.08/1,000	Encephalocele	
0.17–0.15/1,000	Hydrocephalus	
1/1,000 births	Anencephaly	Shija and Kingo, 1985
0.8/1,000 births	Spina bifida	

*f*Births with NTDs were from Princess Badia's, Princess Rashid Teaching Hospital, and other health facilities.
*g*Latin American Collaborative Study of Congenital Malformations.
*h*Metropolitan Atlanta Congenital Defects Program.
*i*Italian Multi-centric Register of Congenital Malformations.
*j*Maternal and Child Health Department of the Ministry of Health.
*k*Korean Federation of Medical Insurance.

TABLE A-10   Studies on the Prevalence of Congenital Heart Disease (CHD)

Country	Year	Population
Africa		
Tunisia	1983–1984	Births, Wassila Bourgiba Hospital, Tunis (live births 9,662, stillbirths 238) (n = 10,000)
Egypt	1990–1991	Children, aged 6–12 yr, 14 schools, Menoufia (n = 8,000)
South Africa	1986–1989	Live births, Kalafong Hospital, Pretoria (n = 17,351)
Asia		
Thailand	1971–1973	Children, aged 4–16 yr, 5 schools, Bang Pa-in, Ayutthaya (n = 2,764)
China	1997	Children, aged 0–2 yr, 13 counties, Zhejing (n = 115,836)
Indonesia	1983–1987	Births, Gunung Wenang Hospital Manado, Jakarta (n = 13,354)
Pakistan	1984	Births (n = 1,134)
India	2001	Random sample of children under 15 yr in Delhi, India (n = 11,833)

Method	Prevalence	Reference
Physical examination within 24 hours of birth	1.3/1,000[a]	Khrouf et al., 1986

Physical examination Tests used to confirm clinically suspected cases:
  Chest X-ray
  Electrocardiography
  Echocardiography
  Color Doppler
	2.6/1,000[b]	Refat et al., 1994

Physical examination within 24 hours of delivery	1.8/1,000 live births	Delport et al., 1995

Physical examination Tests used to confirm clinically suspected cases:
  Chest X-ray
  Electrocardiography
  Cardiac catheterization
	3.3/1,000	Pongpanich et al., 1976

Physical examination Test used to confirm clinically suspected cases: Echocardiography	3.7/1,000 live births	Zhang et al., 1990
Physical examination at birth Test used to confirm clinically suspected cases: Cardiac examination	0.4/1,000 births	Masloman et al., 1991
Physical examination within 1 week of birth	6.2/1,000 births[c]	Jalil et al., 1993
Clinical history or clinical examination	4.2/1,000	Chadha et al., 2001

TABLE A-10   continued

Country	Year	Population
India	1989–1992	Births, Jimper Hospital, Pondicherry (live births 12,337, stillbirths 460) (n = 12,797)
India	1985–1986	Births, Mahatma Gandhi Institute of Medical Sciences, Wardha, Maharashtra (n = 3,014)
India	Not specified	Randomly selected school children, aged 6–16 yr, Jammu-Tawi (n = 10,263)
India	Not specified	Births, Obstetrics Department, S.N. Medical college, Agra (n = 2,720)
Middle East		
Sultanate of Oman	1994–1996	Live births, Royal Hospital and Sultan Qaboos University, Muscat (n = 139,707)
Latin America		
Brazil	1982–1986	Births, 3 hospitals (n = 10,378)
Latin America[m]	1967–1989	Births, 156 hospitals (n = 2,159,065)

Method	Prevalence	Reference
Physical examination with in 24 hours of birth Autopsy[d]	2/1,000 births 1.9/1,000 live births	Bhat and Babu, 1998
Physical examination within 48 hours of birth	1.6/1,000 births[e] 0.3/1,000 births[f]	Chaturvedi and Banerjee, 1989
Physical examination Tests used to confirm clinically suspected cases: Chest X-ray Electrocardiography Echocardiography	0.8/1,000	Gupta et al., 1992
Physical examination within 48 hours of birth	0.7/1,000 births[g]	Kalra et al., 1984
Physical examination Tests used to confirm clinically suspected cases: Chest X-ray Echocardiography Cardiac catheter Angiography	7.1/1,000[h]	Subramanyan et al., 2000
ECLAMC[i] data	0.2/1,000 births[j] 0.3/1,000 births[k] 0.2/1,000 births[l]	Monteleone-Neto and Castilla, 1994
Physical examination at birth Maternal interview (ECLAMC data)	0.5/1,000 births[n] 0.5/1,000 births[o]	Lopez-Camelo and Orioli, 1996

TABLE A-10   continued

Country	Year	Population
Developed Countries		
Finland	1982–1983	Births (n = 133,000)
South Korea	1993–1994	Infants < 1 yr, Korean Federation of Medical Insurance 1993 (n = 601,376) 1994 (n = 601,459)
United States	1981–1982	Live births, Washington, DC, Baltimore, and 5 counties of Virginia (n = 179,697)
United States	1968–1988 1989–1990	Births, Atlanta (n = 580,952) Births, Atlanta (n = 76,862)
Italy	1986–1989 1990	Births (n = 448,195) Births (n = 91,440)
Australia	1981–1984	Live births, Australian Bureau of Statistics, Sydney (n = 343,521)
Canada	1981–1984	Live births, northern and central Alberta (n = 103,411)

Method	Prevalence	Reference
Data source[p] Physical examination Tests used to confirm clinically suspected cases: Echocardiography Cardiac catheterization at operation or necropsy	8.10/1,000 births[q]	Tikkanen and Heinonen, 1992
Data source[r]		Jung et al., 1999
	1993 15.6/1,000 births 1994 14/1,000 births	
Medical records[s]	3.7/1,000 births[t]	Ferencz et al., 1985
MACDP[u] data	0.2/1,000 births[v]	Khoury et al., 1993
IPIMC[w] data	0.8/1,000 births[w]	Khoury et al., 1993
Data source[x]	4.3/1,000 live births	Kidd et al., 1993
Data source[y] physical examination Tests used to confirm clinically suspected cases: Echocardiography Cardiac catheterization at operation or necropsy	Using invasive criteria only 3.4/1,000 births[z] Using noninvasive criteria 5.5/1,000 births	Gabritz et al., 1988

TABLE A-10 continued

Country	Year	Population
Israel	1980–1984	Live births, 1984 (*n* = 86,833)

*a*Type of CHD not specified.

*b*Ventricular septal defect (VSD), pulmonary stenosis (PS), atrial septal defect (ASD), aortic stenosis (AS), mitral valve prolapse (MVP), patent ductus arteriosus (PDA).

*c*5 cases of VSD, 1 case of PS and 1 case Fallot's tetralogy.

*d*Of stillbirths and neonatal deaths with parental consent.

*e*VSD.

*f*Bradyarrhythmia.

*g*Acyanotic and cyanotic CHD.

*h*VSD, ASD, PDA, atrioventricular septal defect (AVSD), PS, AS, coarctation of aorta, tetralogy of Fallot, transposition of great arteries, and miscellaneous others.

*i*Latin American Collaborative Study of Congenital Malformations.

*j*Heart defects, unspecified.

*k*Septal defects.

*l*PDA.

*m*Argentina, Bolivia, Brazil, Chile, Colombia, Peru, and Venezuela.

*n*Heart defect, unspecified.

*o*VSD.

*p*Finnish register of congenital malformations or children's cardiac register.

*q*VSD, ASD, PDA, coarctation of aorta, transposition of great arteries, conus arterious syndrome, hypoplastic left ventricles, endocardial cushion defect, truncus arteriosus, and other rare diseases.

Method	Prevalence	Reference
Data source[aa]	Total 3.5/1,000 Suspected heart defect 1.6/1,000	Kalir, 1985

[r]Korean Federation Medical Insurance.
[s]Collaboration of 5 pediatric cardiology centers and 52 community hospitals, including neonatal and infant deaths.
[t]Transposition of great vessels, tetralogy of Fallot, double outlet right ventricle, truncus arterious, endocardial cushion defect, atresias, valve and vessel lesions, septal defects, and others.
[u]Metropolitan Atlanta Congenital Defects Program.
[v]Cardiac defects include common truncus, transposition of great vessels, tetralogy of Fallot, single ventricle, tricuspid atresia, and hypoplastic left heart.
[w]Italian Multi-centric Register of Congenital Malformations.
[x]Cardiologist records, children's hospital records, autopsy records, and death certificates.
[y]The Heritage Pediatric Cardiology Program, northern and central Alberta.
[z]Transposition of great vessels, tetralogy of Fallot, double outlet right ventricle, PDA, ASD, VSD, AVSD, total anomalous pulmonary venous return, right-sided and left-sided obstructive lesions, complex lesions and others.
[aa]Maternal and Child Health Department of the Ministry of Health.

TABLE A-11 Studies on the Prevalence of Cleft Lip and/or Cleft Palate

Country	Year	Population
Africa		
South Africa	1976–1977	Births (n = 29,633)

Southern
Africa
	1983–1984	Births, Western Cape[a]
		    Whites 10,214
		    Coloreds 31,708
		    Blacks 9,377
		(n = 51,299)

South Africa	1986–1989	Live births, Kalafong Hospital, Pretoria (n = 17,351)
South Africa	1989–1992	Live births, Mankweng Hospital, Sovenga, Northern Transvaal (n = 7,617)
Tunisia	1983–1984	Births, Wassila Bourgiba Hospital, Tunis (live births 9,662, stillbirths 238) (n = 10,000)
Zimbabwe	1984	Births, Harare Maternity Hospital and clinics, Greater Harare (n = 18,033) Neonatal admissions (n = 2,154)
Uganda	1956–1957	Births, Mulago Hospital, Kampala (live births 1,927, stillbirths 141) (n = 2,068)
Zaire	1977–1979	Live births, Mama Yerno Hospital (n = 56,637)
Asia		
Philippines	1989–1996	Births, 6 cities[e] (n = 47,969)
China	1980–1989	Live births, 22 Shanghai hospitals (n = 541,504)

Method	Prevalence	Reference
Birth records from pediatric ward and mortuary	Facial cleft 0.30/1,000 births	Kromberg and Jenkins, 1982
Data source [b] Physical examination of infants, age <1 yr	Total 1/1,000 births Whites 0.6/1,000 births Coloreds 1.4/1,000 births Blacks 0.3/1,000 births	Morrison et al., 1985
Physical examination within 24 hours of birth	CL & CP[c] 0.12/1,000 live births	Delport et al., 1995
Physical examination within 24 hours of birth	CL/CP[d] 0.4/1,000 live births	Venter, 1995
Physical examination within 24 hours of birth	CL/CP 0.4/1,000 births CL 0.6/1,000 births CP 0.4/1,000 births	Khrouf et al., 1986
Hospital records	CL/CP 0.3/1,000 births	Shija and Kingo, 1985
Physical examination at birth	CL 0.5/1,000 births CL & CP 1/1,000 births	Simpkiss and Lowe, 1961
Hospital records	All clefts 0.5/1,000 live births CL/CP 0.4/1,000 live births	Ogle, 1993
CLMMRH[f] medical records	CL/CP 1.9/1,000 births	Murray et al., 1997
Hospital records 1980–1986 Physical examination at birth 1987–1989	CL/CP 1.2/1,000 births	Cooper et al., 2000

TABLE A-11   continued

Country	Year	Population
China	1986–1987	Births, 945 hospitals in 29 provinces (live and stillbirths) ($n = 1,243,284$)
China	1988–1991	Births, National Center for Birth Defects Monitoring ($n = 2,750,588$)
China	1985–1987	Births, 30 hospitals, Anhui province ($n = 46,811$)
Indonesia	1983–1987	Births, Gunung Wenang Hospital, Manado, Jakarta ($n = 13,354$)
India	1989–1992	Births, Jimper Hospital, Pondicherry (live births 12,337 stillbirths 460) ($n = 12,797$)
India	1985–1986	Births, Mahatma Gandhi Institute of Medical Sciences, Wardha, Maharashtra ($n = 3,014$)
India	1976–1987	Births, 5 hospitals, West Bengal, ($n = 115,851$)
	1986–1987	Births, Malda Sadar Hospital, West Bengal ($n = 10,415$)
India	Not specified	Births, Obstetrics Department, S.N. Medical College, Agra ($n = 2,720$)
Middle East Saudi Arabia	1989–1992	Live births, Health ministry of Central Province ($n = 62,557$)

Method	Prevalence	Reference
Hospital records	CL & CP 1.3–3.1/1,000 births Average 1.8/1,000 births Rural 2.1/1,000 births Urban 1.7/1,000 births	Xiao, et al., 1989
Hospital records	CL & CP 11–26/1,000 births	Wu et al., 1995
Hospital records	CL & CP 2.5/1,000 births	Shi, 1989
Physical examination at birth	CL & CP 0.9/1,000 births	Masloman et al., 1991
Physical examination within 24 hours of birth Autopsy[g]	CL/CP 1.95/1,000 births	Bhat and Babu,1998
Physical examination within 48 hours of birth	CL/CP 2.3/1,000 births	Chaturvedi and Banerjee, 1989
Hospital records [h]	CL/CP 0.7/1,000 live births	Choudhury et al., 1989
Physical examination	CL/CP 1/1,000 live births	
Physical examination within 48 hours of birth	CL 2.5/1,000 births CP 1.5/1,000 births	Kalra et al., 1984
Hospital records,[i] 1989–1990 Physical examination at birth, 1990–1992	CL & CP 2.2/1,000 live births CL/CP 1.9/1,000 live births CL 0.9/1,000 live births CP 0.3/1,000 live births	Borkar et al., 1993

TABLE A-11 continued

Country	Year	Population
Saudi Arabia	1982–1988	Live births, King Khalid University Hospital, Riyadh (n = 20,045)
Iran	1976–1991	Live births, Maternity Hospital, Shiraz (n = 19,369)
Latin America		
Latin American Study	1967–1989	Hospital births (n = 2,159,065)
Argentina		
Brazil		
Chile		
Venezuela		
Colombia		
Peru		
Bolivia		
Latin America	1967–1992	Live births (n = 2,876,686)
Spain	1976–1993	Live births (n = 1,074,029)

Method	Prevalence	Reference
Hospital records[j]	Facial clefts 0.3/1,000 live births	Kumar et al., 1991
Hospital records	Total clefts 1/1,000 live births CL/CP 0.6/1,000 live births CP 0.4/1,000 live births	Rajabian and Sherkat, 2000
ECLAMC[k] data	Prevalence of cleft lip Buenos Aires 1.3/1,000 births Central 1.2/1,000 births Patagonia 1.6/1,000 births Northeast 0.9/1,000 births Southeast 0.8/1,000 births South 1.1/1,000 births Central 1.2/1,000 births South 1.4/1,000 births 0.8/1,000 births Savana 0.8/1,000 births Sierra 1/1,000 births 0.7/1,000 births Altiplano 2.5/1,000	Lopez-Camelo and Orioli, 1996
ECLAMC data	Total clefts 1.4/1,000 live births CL/CP 0.8/1,000 live births CP 0.6/1,000 live births	Castilla and Martinez- Frias, 1995
ECEMC[l] data	Total clefts 1.1/1,000 live births CL/CP 0.6/1,000 live births CP 0.5/1,000 live births	Castilla and Martinez Frias, 1995

TABLE A-11 continued

Country	Year	Population
South America[m]	1967–1981	Births, 56 hospitals in 8 countries (n = 849,381)
Developed Countries		
Japan	1994–1995	Live births, 1,532 maternity institutions (n = 303,738)
Singapore	1986–1988	Live births, Kandang Kerbau Hospital (n = 30,411)
United States	1968–1988	Births, Atlanta (n = 580,952)
	1989–1990	Births, Atlanta (n = 76,862)
Sweden	1991–1995	Live births,[o] Stockholm (n = 122,148)
Italy	1986–1989	Births (n = 448,195)
	1990	Births (n = 91,440)
Israel	1980–1984	Live births, 1984 (n = 86,833)

Method	Prevalence	Reference
ECLAMC data	CL/CP 0.9/1,000 births	Menegotto and Salzano, 1991
Questionnaire	CL/CP 1.4/1,000 live births	Natsume et al., 2000

Physical examination
at birth
	Facial clefts
	1.7/1,000 live births
	  Chinese 2/1,000 live
	  births
	  Malays 1.4/1,000 live
	  births
	  Indians 0.9/1,000 live
	  births
		Tan, 1988

MACDP[n] data	CL/CP 1/1,000 births CP 0.5/1,000 births	Khoury et al., 1993

Hospital records
Parental interviews
	CL & CP
	2/1,000 live births
	  CL
	  0.4/1,000 live births
	  CP
	  0.7/1,000 live births
	CL/CP
	0.7/1,000 live births
		Hagberg et al.,
		1998

IPIMC[p] data	CL/CP 0.6/1,000 births CP 0.5/1,000 births	Khoury et al., 1993
Data source[q]	CP 0.3/1,000 live births CL 0.2/1,000 live births CL & CP 0.3/1,000 live births	Kalir, 1985

TABLE A-11 continued

Country	Year	Population
Argentina	1967–1995	Births, 53 hospitals (n = 1,668,733)

[a]Greater Cape Town, Bellville, Paarl, Stellenbosch, Somerset West, Wellington, Wynberg, Simonstown, Kuilsriver, and Goodwood.
[b]Tygerberg and Red Cross Memorial Children's Hospital and plastic surgeons in private practice.
[c]CL&CP, cleft lip and cleft palate.
[d]CL/CP, cleft lip with or without cleft palate.
[e]Manila, Lucena, Naga, Bacolod, Iligan and Davao city.
[f]Pediatric Department of Corazon Locsin Montelibano Memorial Regional Hospital.
[g]Includes stillbirths and neonatal deaths with parental consent.
[h]National Medical College, Matri Mangal Seva Prathisthan, Sishu Mangal Seva

Method	Prevalence	Reference
ECLAMC data	Lowland CP 0.2/1,000 births CL 0.9/1,000 births Highland CP 0.2/1,000 births CL 1.7/1,000 births	Castilla et.al., 1999

Pratisthan, Chinsurah Sadar Hospital, Baharampur Sadar Hospital, and Malda Sadar Hospital.
[i]King Fahd Specialist Hospital, Buraidah.
[j]Plastic Surgery Division of King Khalid University Hospital to which all cleft lip or cleft palate cases are referred.
[k]Latin American Collaborative Study of Congenital Malformations.
[l]Spanish Collaborative Study of Congenital Malformations.
[m]Uruguay, Chile, Argentina, Brazil, Bolivia, Ecuador, Venezuela
[n]Metropolitan Atlanta Congenital Defects Program.
[o]20% of all live births in Sweden.
[p]Italian Multi-centric Register of Congenital Malformations.
[q]Maternal and Child Health Department, Ministry of Health.

TABLE A-12   Studies on the Prevalence of Talipes

Country	Year	Population
Africa		
South Africa	1986–1989	Live births, Kalafong Hospital, Pretoria (n = 17,351)
South Africa	1976–1977	Births (n = 29,633)
Tunisia	1983–1984	Births, Wassila Bourgiba Hospital, Tunis (live births 9662, stillbirths 238) (n = 10,000)
Uganda	1956–1957	Births, Mulago Hospital, Kampala (live 1927, still 141) (n = 2,068)
Latin America		
Latin America[a]	1967–1989	Births (n = 2,159,065)
South America[a]	1967–1978	Births, 59 maternity hospitals (n = 671,494)
South America[d]	1982–1988	Births (n = 869,750)
Argentina	1967–1995	Births (n = 1,668,733)
Brazil	1982–1986	Births, 3 hospitals (n = 10,378)
Asia		
Malaysia	1988	Births, Maternity Hospital, Kuala Lumpur (n = 8,369)

Method	Prevalence	Reference
Physical examination within 24 hours of birth	0.5/1,000 live births	Delport et al., 1995
Data, pediatric ward and mortuary records	1.55/1,000 births	Kromberg and Jenkins, 1982
Physical examination within 24 hours of birth	2.6/1,000 births	Khrouf et al., 1986
Physical examination at birth	0.5/1,000 births	Simpkiss and Lowe, 1961
ECLAMC[b] data	1.8/1,000 births	Lopez-Camelo and Orioli, 1996
ECLAMC data physical examination at birth	0.4/1,000 births	Nunes and Dutra, 1986
ECLAMC data	1.8/1,000 births	Castilla and Lopez Camelo, 1990
ECLAMC data physical examination at birth	Lowland Equinovarus 1.1/1,000 Talgovarus 0.2/1,000 Highland Equinovarus 0.6/1,000 Talgovarus 0.2/1,000	Castilla et al., 1999
ECLAMC data	1.7/1,000 births	Monteleone-Neto and Castilla, 1994
Physical examination at birth	5.6/1,000 births 4.5/1,000 births[e] 1.3/1,000 births[f]	Boo and Ong, 1990

TABLE A-12 continued

Country	Year	Population
Thailand	1975–1977	Births, Chulalongkorn hospital, Bangkok (n = not specified)
Indonesia	1983–1987	Births, Gunung Wenang Hospital Manado, Jakarta (n = 13,354)
India	1980–1984	Live births (n = 13,321)
India	1976–1987	Births, 5 hospitals West Bengal (n = 115,851)
	1986–1987	Births, Malda Sadar Hospital, West Bengal (n = 10,415)
India	1976–1980	Births, National Medical College Hospital, Calcutta (n = 21,016)
India	1989–1992	Births, Jimper Hospital, Pondicherry (live births 12,337, stillbirths 460) (n = 12,797)
India	Not specified	Births, Obstetrics Department, S.N. Medical College, Agra (n = 2,720)
India	1985–1986	Births, Mahatma Gandhi Institute of Medical Sciences, Wardha, Maharashtra (n = 3,014)

[a]Argentina, Bolivia, Brazil, Chile, Colombia, Peru, Venezuela.
[b]Latin American Collaborative Study of Congenital Malformations.
[c]Argentina, Brazil, Chile, Equador, Peru, Uruguay, Venezuela.
[d]South American countries, plus Costa Rica and Dominican Republic.
[e]Congenital talipes equinovarus.
[f]Congenital talipes calcaneovalgus.
[g]National Medical college, Matri Mangal Seva Prathisthan, Sishu Mangal Seva Pratisthan, Chinsurah Sadar Hospital, Bahararnpur Sadar Hospital, and Malda Sadar Hospital.
[h]Includes stillbirths and neonatal deaths with parental consent.

Method	Prevalence	Reference
Hospital records	1.3/1,000 live births	Limpaphayom and Jirachaiprasit, 1985
Physical examination at birth	0.8/1,000 births	Masloman et al., 1991
Examination of infants after birth	1.6/1,000 live births	Bahadur and Bhat, 1989
Hospital records[g]	0.6/1,000 births	Choudhury et al., 1989
Physical examination		
Hospital records	0.3/1,000 births	Choudhury et al., 1984
Physical examination within 24 hours of birth Autopsy[h]	2/1,000 births	Bhat and Babu, 1998
Physical examination within 48 hours of birth	1.5/1,000 births	Kalra et al., 1984
Physical examination within 48 hours of birth	1/1,000 births	Chaturvedi and Banerjee, 1989

TABLE A-13   Studies of the Prevalence of Developmental Dysplasia of
the Hip (DDH)

Country	Year	Population
Africa		
South Africa	1986–1989	Live births, Kalafong Hospital, Pretoria (*n* = 17,351)
Tunisia	1983–1984	Births, Wassila Bourgiba Hospital, Tunis (live births 9,662, stillbirths 238) (*n* = 10,000)
Asia		
Malaysia	1984–1987	Live births, Alor Setar General Hospital (*n* = 19,769)
Pakistan	1984	Births (*n* = 1,134)
India	1989–1990	Hospital births in urban community (*n* = 6,029)
India	1989–1992	Births, Jimper Hospital, Pondicherry (live births 12,337, stillbirths 460) (*n* = 12,797)
Middle East and Eastern Europe		
Saudia Arabia	1991–1993	Live births, King Fahd Hofuf Hospital (*n* = 30,159)
Hungary	1970–1980s	Not specified

Method	Prevalence	Reference
Physical examination within 24 hours of birth	0.06/1,000 births	Delport et al., 1995
Physical examination within 24 hours of birth	Hip instability 4.1/1,000 births	Khrouf et al., 1986
Physical examination within 48 hours of birth Tests used to confirm clinically suspected cases: Lab investigations, Ultrasound, radiological, cardiac, neurological examination	0.2/1,000 births	Peng and Chuan, 1988
Physical examination within 1 week of birth	1/1,134 births 0.9/1,000 births	Jalil et al., 1993
Physical examination Ortolani and Barlow provocative tests Test used to confirm clinically suspected cases: Ultrasonography Radiological evaluation	Unstable 18.7/1,000 births Subluxatable hips 12.1/1,000 births Dislocated hips 0.8/1,000 births	Gupta et al., 1992
Physical examination within 24 hours of birth Autopsy[a]	0.3/1,000 births	Bhat and Babu, 1998
Hospital records	0.4/1,000 live births	Refat et al., 1995
Data source[b]	13.62/1,000	Czeizel et al., 1993

TABLE A-13 continued

Country	Year	Population
Lebanon	1991–1993	Births (n = 3,865)
Latin America South America[c]	1982–1986	Births (n = 869,750)
Brazil	1982–1985	Births, 3 maternity hospitals,[e] Cubatao (n = 10,378)
Latin American Study Argentina	1967–1989	Hospital births (n = 2,159,065)
Brazil	1967–1989	Hospital births
Chile	1967–1989	Hospital births
Venezuela	1967–1989	Hospital births
Colombia	1967–1989	Hospital births
Peru	1967–1989	Hospital births
Bolivia	1967–1989	Hospital births

Method	Prevalence	Reference
Physical examination within 24 hours of birth Test used to confirm clinically suspected cases: Radiography	1.8/1,000 births	Bittar, 1995
ECLAMC data[d]	Hip subdislocation 2.1/1,000 Hip dislocation 0.2/1,000	Castilla and Lopez-Camelo, 1990
ECLAMC data Physical examination at birth	1.8/1,000 births	Monteleone-Neto and Castilla, 1994
ECLAMC data	Buenos Aires 0.4/1,000 births Central 0.3/1,000 births Patagonia 0.7/1,000 births	Lopez Camelo and Orioli, 1996
ECLAMC data	Northeast 0.03/1,000 births Southeast 0.3/1,000 births South 0.2/1,000 births	Lopez-Camelo and Orioli, 1996
ECLAMC data	Central 0.1/1,000 births South 0.01/1,000 births	Lopez-Camelo and Orioli, 1996
ECLAMC data	0.1/1,000 births	Lopez-Camelo and Orioli, 1996
ECLAMC data	Savana 0.1/1,000 births Sierra 0.2/1,000 births	Lopez-Camelo and Orioli, 1996
ECLAMC data	0.2/1,000 births	Lopez-Camelo and Orioli, 1996
ECLAMC data	Altiplano 0.04/1,000 births	Lopez-Camelo and Orioli, 1996

TABLE A-13   continued

Country	Year	Population
Developed Countries		
Hong Kong	1960–1975	Births, Sandy Bay Children's Hospital
	1968	(n = 82,992)
	1974	(n = 81,879)
Israel	1980–1984	Births
	1980	(n = 85,575)
	1984	(n = 86,833)
South Korea	1993–1994	Infants <1 yr, Korean Federation of Medical Insurance (KFMI)
	1993	(n = 601,376)
	1994	(n = 601,459)

[a]Includes stillbirths and neonatal deaths with parental consent.
[b]Hungarian Congenital Abnormality Registry and Medical Records, all institutions.
[c]12 Latin American countries: 10 South American countries plus Costa Rica and Dominican Republic.
[d]Latin American Collaborative Study of Congenital Malformations.
[e]Oswaldo Cruz, Ana Costa, and De Cubatao.
[f]Maternal and Child Health Department of the Ministry of Health.

Method	Prevalence	Reference
In-patients' and outpatients' hospital records	1968 0.1/1,000 births 1974 0.1/1,000 births	Hoaglund et al., 1981
Data source*f*	1980 3.3/1,000 births 1984 2.8/1,000 births	Kalir, 1985
Data from KFMI	1993 1.1/1,000 infants 1994 0.9/1,000 infants	Jung et al., 1999

REFERENCES

Adeyokunnu AA. 1982. The incidence of Down syndrome in Nigeria. *Journal of Medical Genetics* 19(4):277–279.

Airede KI. 1992. Neural tube defects in the middle belt of Nigeria. *Journal of Tropical Pediatrics* 38(1):27–30.

Aksu TA, Essen F, Dolunay MS, Aliciguzel Y, Yucel G, Cali S, Baykal Y. 1990. Erythrocyte glucose-6-phosphate dehydrogenase (1.1.1.49) deficiency in Antalya Province, Turkey: An epidemiologic and biochemical study. *American Journal of Epidemiology* 131(6): 1094–1097.

Al-Awadi SA, Farage TI, Teebi AS, Naguib KK, Sundareshan TS, Murthy DS. 1990. Down syndrome in Kuwait. *American Journal of Medical Genetics* 7(suppl):87–88.

Al-Mahroos F. 1998. Cystic fibrosis in Bahrain: Incidence, phenotype and outcome. *Journal of Tropical Pediatrics* 44(1):35–39.

Al-Naama MM, al-Naama LM, al-Sadoon TA. 1994. Glucose-6-phosphate dehydrogenase, hexokinase and pyruvate kinase activities in erythrocytes of neonates and adults in Basrah. *Annals of Tropical Pediatrics* 14(3):195–200.

Amin-Zaki L, el-Din ST, Kubba B. 1972. Glucose-6-phosphate dehydrogenase deficiency among ethnic groups in Iraq. *Bulletin of the World Health Organization* 47(1):1–5.

Angastiniotis MA, Hadjiminas MG. 1981. Prevention of thalassaemia in Cyprus. *Lancet* 1(8216):369–371.

Angastiniotis M, Modell B, Englezos P, Boulyjenkov V. 1995. Prevention and control of haemoglobinopathies. *Bulletin of the World Health Organization* 73(3):375–386.

Aquaron R. 1990. Oculocutaneous albinism in Cameroon: A 15-year follow-up study. *Ophthalmic Paediatric Genetics* 11(4):255–263.

Bahadur RA, Bhat BV. 1989. Congenital musculoskeletal malformations in neonates. *Journal of the Indian Medical Association* 87(2):27–29.

Balgir RS, Murmu B, Dash BP. 1999. Hereditary hemolytic disorders among the Ashram school children in Mayurbhanj district of Orissa. *Journal of the Association of Physicians of India* 47(10):987–990.

Barnicot NA. 1952. Albinism in South Western Nigeria. *Annals of Human Genetics* 17:38–72.

Bashir N, Barkawi M, Sharif L. 1991. Prevalence of haemoglobinopathies in school children in Jordan Valley. *Annals of Tropical Pediatrics* 11(4):373–376.

Bashir N, Barkawi M, Sharif L, Momani A, Gharaibeh N. 1992. Prevalence of hemoglobinopathies in north Jordan. *Tropical and Geographical Medicine* 44(1–2):122–125.

Bhat BV, Babu L. 1998. Congenital malformations at birth: A prospective study from south India. *Indian Journal of Pediatrics* 65(6):873–881.

Bittar Z. 1995. Major anomalies in consecutive births in south Beirut: A preliminary report about incidence of pattern. *Le Journal Médical Libanais* 43(2):62–67.

Bittar Z. 1998. Major congenital malformations presenting in the first 24 hours of life in 3865 consecutive births in south of Beirut. Incidence and pattern. *Le Journal Médical Libanais* 46(5):256–260.

Boo NY, Ong LC. 1990. Congenital talipes in Malaysian neonates: Incidence, pattern and associated factors. *Singapore Medical Journal* (6):539–542.

Boo NY, Hoe TS, Lye MS, Poon PK, Mahani MC. 1989. Maternal age-specific incidence of Down's syndrome in Malaysian neonates. *Journal of the Singapore Paediatric Society* 31(3–4):138–142.

Borkar AS, Mathur AK, Mahaluxmivala S. 1993. Epidemiology of facial clefts in the central province of Saudi Arabia. *British Journal of Plastic Surgery* 46(8):673–675.

Bouma MJ, Goris M, Akhtar T, Khan N, Khan N, Kita E. 1995. Prevalence and clinical presentation of glucose-6-phosphate dehydrogenase deficiency in Pakistani Pathan and Afghan refugee communities in Pakistan: Implications for the use of primaquine in regional malaria control programmes. *Transactions of the Royal Society of Tropical Medicine and Hygiene* 89(1):62–64.

Buccimazza SS, Molteno CD, Dunne TT, Viljoen DL. 1994. Prevalence of neural tube defects in Cape Town, South Africa. *Teratology* 50(3):194–199.

Cao A, Rosatelli C, Pirastu M, Galanello R. 1991.Thalassemias in Sardinia: Molecular pathology phenotype-genotype correlation and prevention. *American Journal of Pediatric Hematology/Oncology* 13(2):179–188.

Castilla EE, Lopez-Camelo JS. 1990. The surveillance of birth defects in South America: I. The search for time clusters: Epidemics. *Advances in Mutagenesis Research* 2:191–210.

Castilla EE, Martinez-Frias M. 1995. Congenital healed cleft lip. *American Journal of Medical Genetics* 58(2):106–112.

Castilla EE, Lopez-Camelo JS, Campaña H. 1999. Altitude as a risk factor for congenital anomalies. *American Journal of Medical Genetics* 86(1):9–14.

Chadha SL, Singh N, Shukla DK. 2001. Epidemiological study of congenital heart disease. *Indian Journal of Pediatrics* 68(6):507–510.

Chaturvedi P, Banerjee KS. 1989. Spectrum of congenital malformations in the newborns from Rural Maharashtra. *Indian Journal of Pediatrics* 56(4):501–507.

Chaturvedi P, Banerjee KS. 1993. An epidemiological study of congenital malformations in newborn. *Indian Journal of Pediatrics* 60(5):645–653.

Chiang SH, Wu SJ, Wu KF, Hsiao KJ. 1999. Neonatal screening for glucose-6-phosphate dehydrogenase deficiency in Taiwan. *Southeast Asian Journal of Tropical Medicine and Public Health* 30(suppl 2):72–74.

Choudhury A, Talukder G, Sharma A. 1984. Neonatal congenital malformations in Calcutta. *Indian Pediatrics* 21(5):399–405.

Choudhury AR, Mukherjee M, Sharma A, Talukder G, Ghosh PK. 1989. Study of 1,26,266 consecutive births for major congenital defects. *Indian Journal of Pediatrics* 56(4):493–499.

Cin S, Akar N, Arcasoy A, Dedeoglu S, Cavdar AO. 1984. Prevalence of thalassemia and G6PD deficiency in North Cyprus. *Acta Haematology* 71(1):69–70.

Collaborative Study. 1975. Frequency of inborn errors of metabolism, especially PKU, in some representative newborn screening centers around the world: A collaborative study. *Humangenetik* 30(4):273–286.

Cooper ME, Stone RA, Liu Y, Hu DN, Melnick M, Marazita ML. 2000. Descriptive epidemiology of nonsyndromic cleft lip with or without cleft palate in Shanghai, China, from 1980 to 1989. *Cleft Palate-Craniofacial Journal* 37(3):274–280.

Crowther C, Glyn-Jones R. 1986. Lethal congenital malformations in the Greater Harare Obstetric Unit during 1983. *Central African Journal of Medicine* 32(2):39, 41–43.

Czeizel AE. 1997. First 25 years of the Hungarian congenital abnormality registry. *Teratology* 55(5):229–305.

Czeizel AE, Intody Z, Modell B. 1993. What proportion of congenital abnormalities can be prevented? *British Medical Journal* 306(6880):499–503.

Daoud AS, Al-Kaysi F, El-Shanti H, Batieha A, Obeidat A, Al-Sheyyab M. 1997. *Saudi Medical Journal* 17(1):78–81.

Delport SD, Christianson AL, van den Berg HJ, Wolmarans L, Gericke GS. 1995. Congenital anomalies in black South African liveborn neonates at an urban academic hospital. *South African Medical Journal* 85(1):11–15.

El-Hazmi MA, Warsy AS, al-Swailem AR, Al-Swailem A, Bahakim HM. 1996. Sickle cell gene in the population of Saudi Arabia. *Hemoglobin* 20(3):187–198.

Fan GX, Jun Y, Rui-guan C. 1999. Neonatal screening of phenylketonuria and congenital hypothyroidism in China. *Southeast Asian Journal of Tropical Medicine and Public Health* 30(suppl 2):17–19.

Farhud DD, Kabiri M. 1982. Incidence of phenylketonuria (PKU) in Iran. *Indian Journal of Pediatrics* 49(400):685–688.

Ferencz C, Rubin JD, McCarter RJ, Brenner JI, Neill CA, Perry LW, Hepner SI, Downing JW. 1985. Congenital heart disease: Prevalence at live birth. The Baltimore-Washington infant study. *American Journal of Epidemiology* 121(1):31–36.

Fok TF, Lau SP, Fung KP. 1985. Cord blood G-6-PD activity by quantitative enzyme assay and fluorescent spot test in Chinese neonates. *Australian Paediatric Journal* 21(1):23–25.

Gabritz RG, Joffres MR, Collins-Nakai RL. 1988. Congenital heart disease: Incidence in the first year of life. The Alberta Heritage Pediatric Cardiology Program. *American Journal of Epidemiology* 128(2):381–388.

Ganeshaguru K, Acquaye JK, Samuel AP, Hassounah F, Agyeiobese S, Azrai LM, Sejeny SA, A Omer. 1987. Prevalence of thalassaemias in ethnic Saudi Arabians. *Tropical and Geographical Medicine* 39(3):238–243.

Granda H, Gispert S, Martinez G, Gomez M, Ferreira R, Collazo T, Magarino C, Heredero L. 1994. Results from a reference laboratory for prenatal diagnosis of sickle cell disorders in Cuba. *Prenatal Diagnosis* 14(8):659–662.

Gupta I, Gupta ML, Parihar A, Gupta CD. 1992. Epidemiology of rheumatic and congenital heart disease in school children. *Journal of the Indian Medical Association* 90(3):57–59.

Gurson CT, Sertel H, Gurkan M, Pala S. 1973. Newborn screening for cystic fibrosis with the chloride electrode and neutron activation analysis. *Helvetica Paediatrica Acta* 28(2):165–174.

Hagberg C, Larson O, Milerad J. 1998. Incidence of cleft lip palate and risks of additional malformations. *Cleft Palate–Craniofacial Journal* 35(1):40–45.

Harris RG, Prieto L. 1925. The scientific importance of the White Indians. *World's Work* 49:211–217.

Himmetoglu O, Tiras MB, Gursoy R, Karabacak O, Sahin I, Onan A. 1996. The incidence of congenital malformations in a Turkish populations. *International Journal of Gynaecology and Obstetrics* 55(2):117–121.

Hitzeroth HW, Niehaus CE, Brill DC. 1995. Phenylketonuria in South Africa. A report on the status quo. *South African Medical Journal* 85(1):33–36.

Hoaglund FT, Kalamchi A, Poon R, Chow SP, Yau AC. 1981. Congenital hip dislocation and dysplasia in Southern Chinese. *International Orthopaedics* 4(4):243–246.

Hoe TS, Boo NY, Clyde MM. 1989. Incidence of Down's syndrome in a large Malaysian maternity hospital over an 18-month period. *Singapore Medical Journal* 30(3):246–248.

Hosani HA, Czeizel AE. 2000. Congenital abnormalities in the United Arab Emirates. *Teratology* 61(3):161–162.

Hu YH, Li LM, Li P. 1996. A five years surveillance on neural system birth defects in rural areas of China [Article in Chinese]. *Zhonghua Liu Xing Bing Xue Za Zhi* 17(1):20–24.

Imaizumi Y, Yamamura H, Nishikawa M, Matsuoka M, Moriyama I. 1991. The prevalence of birth congenital malformations at a maternity hospital in Osaka City, 1948–1990. *Jinrui Idengaku Zasshi (Japanese Journal of Human Genetics)* 36(3):275–287.

Isaac GS, Krishnamurty PS, Reddy YR, Ahuja YR. 1985. Down's syndrome in Hyderabad, India. *Acta Anthropogenetica* 9(4):256–260.

Jalil F, Lindblad BS, Hanson LA, Khan SR, Yaqoob M, Karlberg J. 1993. Early child health in Lahore, Pakistan: IX. Perinatal events. *Acta Paediatrica* 390(suppl):95–107.

Jaovisidha A, Ajjimarkorn S, Panburana P, Somboonsub O, Herabutya Y, Rungsiprakarn R. 2000. Prevention and control of thalassemia in Ramathibodi Hospital, Thailand. *Southeast Asian Journal of Tropical Medicine and Public Health* 31(3):561–565.

Joseph R, Ho LY, Gomez JM, Rajdurai VS, Sivasankaran S, Yip YY. 1999. Mass newborn screening for glucose-6-phospate dehydrogenase deficiency in Singapore. *Southeast Asian Journal of Tropical Medicine and Public Health* 30(suppl 2):70–71.

Jung S-C, Kim S, Yoon, K, Lee J. 1999. Prevalence of congenital malformations and genetic diseases in Korea. *Journal of Human Genetics* 44(1):30–34.

Kagore F, Lund PM. 1995. Oculocutaneous albinism among schoolchildren in Harare, Zimbabwe. *Journal of Medical Genetics* 32(11):859–861.

Kalir A. 1985. A national monitoring system for congenital malformations in Israel. *Israel Journal of Medical Sciences* 21(9):731–736.

Kalra A, Kalra K, Sharma V, Singh M, Dayal RS. 1984. Congenital malformations. *Indian Pediatrics* 21(12):945–950.

Kamble M, Chaturvedi P. 2000. Epidemiology of sickle cell disease in a rural hospital of central India. *Indian Pediatrics* 37(4):391–396.

Kar BC. 1991. Sickle cell disease in India. *Journal of the Association of Physicians of India* 39(12):954–960.

Kate SL. 2000. Health problems of tribal population groups from the State of Maharashtra. *Indian Journal of Medical Science* 55(2):99–108.

Kaur M, Das GP, Verma IC. 1997. Sickle cell trait and disease among tribal communities in Orissa, Madhya Pradesh and Kerala. *Indian Journal of Medical Research* 105:111–116.

Kazmi KA, Rab SM. 1990. Sickle cell anaemia in Pakistan. *British Journal of Clinical Practice* (11):503–555.

Keeler CE. 1964. The incidence of Cuna Moon-child albinos. *Journal of Heredity* 55:155.

Keeler CE. 1970. Cuna Moon-child albinism, 1950–1970. *Journal of Heredity* 61(6):273–278.

Keeler CE, Prieto L. 1950. The Caribe-Cuna Moon-child: A demonstration of pigment-gene pleiotrophy in man. *Bulletin of the Georgia Academy of Science* 8:3–6.

Kerem E, Kalman YM, Yahav V, Shoshani T, Abeliovich D, Szeinberg A, Rivlin J, Blau H, Tal A, Ben-Tur L, Springer C, Augarten A, Godfrey S, Lerer I, Branski D, Friedman M, Kerem B. 1995. Highly variable incidence of cystic fibrosis and different mutation distribution among different Jewish ethnic groups in Israel. *Human Genetics* 96(2):193–197.

Keskin A, Turk T, Polat A, Koyuncu H, Saracoglu B. 2000. Premarital screening of beta-thalassemia trait in the province of Denizli, Turkey. *Acta Haematologica* 104(1):31–33.

Khoury MJ, Botto L, Waters GD, Mastroiacovo P, Castilla E, Erickson JD. 1993. Monitoring for new multiple congenital anomalies in the search for human teratogens. *American Journal of Medical Genetics* 46(4):460–466.

Khrouf N, Spang R, Podgorna T, Miled SB, Moussaoui M, Chibani M. 1986. Malformations in 10,000 consecutive births in Tunis. *Acta Paediatrica Scandinavica* 75(4):534–539.

Kidd SA, Lancaster PA, McCredie RM. 1993. The incidence of congenital heart defects in the first year of life. *Journal of Paediatrics and Child Health* 29(5):344–349.

Kromberg JG, Jenkins T. 1982. Prevalence of albinism in the South African negro. *South African Medical Journal* 61(11):383–386.

Kulkarni ML, Mathew MA, Ramachandran B. 1987. High incidence of neural-tube defects in South India. *Lancet* 1(8544):1260.

Kulkarni ML, Mathew MA, Reddy V. 1989. The range of neural tube defects in southern India. *Archives of Disease in Childhood* 64(2):201–204.

Kumar P, Hussain MT, Cardos E, Hawary MB, Hussanain J. 1991. Facial clefts in Saudi Arabia: An epidemiologic analysis in 179 patients. *Plastic Reconstructive Surgery* 88(6):955–958.

Limpaphayom M, Jirachaiprasit P. 1985. Factors related with the incidence of congenital clubfoot in Thai children. *Journal of the Medical Association of Thailand* 68(1):1–5.

Liu SR, Zuo QH. 1986. Newborn screening for phenylketonuria in eleven districts. *Chinese Medical Journal* 99(2):113–118.

Lopez-Camelo JS, Orioli IM. 1996. Heterogeneous rates for birth defects in Latin America: Hints of causality. *Genetic Epidemiology* 13(5):469–481.

Lugovska R, Vevere P, Andrusaite R, Kornejeva A. 1999. Newborn screening for PKU and congenital hypothyroidism in Latvia. *Southeast Asian Journal of Tropical Medicine and Public Health* 30(suppl 2):52–53.

Lund PM. 1996. Distribution of oculocutaneous albinism in Zimbabwe. *Journal of Medical Genetics* 33(8):641–644.

Lund PM, Puri N, Durham-Pierre D, King RA, Brilliant MH. 1997. Oculocutaneous albinism in an isolated Tonga community in Zimbabwe. *Journal of Medical Genetics* 34(9):733–735.

Masloman N, Mustadjab I, Munir M. 1991. Congenital malformation at Gunung Wenang Hospital Manado: A five-year spectrum. *Paediatrica Indonesiana* 31(11–12):294–302.

Melnick M, Marazita ML. 1998. Neural tube defects, methylenetetrahydrofolate reductase mutation, and north/south dietary differences in China. *Journal of Craniofacial Genetics and Developmental Biology* 18(4):233–235.

Menegotto BG, Salzano FM. 1991. Epidemiology of oral clefts in a large South American sample. *Cleft Palate Craniofacial Journal* 28(4):373–377.

Mir NA, Fakhri M, Abdelaziz M, Kishan J, Elzouki A, Baxi AJ, Sheriff DS, Prasanan KG. 1985. Erythrocyte glucose-6-phosphate dehydrogenase status of newborns and adults in eastern Libya. *Annals of Tropical Paediatrics* 5(4):211–213.

Missiou-Tsagaraki S. 1991. Screening for glucose-6-phosphate dehydrogenase deficiency as a preventive measure: Prevalence among 1,286,000 Greek newborn infants. *Journal of Pediatrics* 119(2):292–299.

Molteno C, Smart R, Viljoen D, Sayed R, Roux A. 1997. Twenty-year birth prevalence of Down syndrome in Cape Town, South Africa. *Paediatric and Perinatal Epidemiology* 11(4):428–435.

Monteleone-Neto R, Castilla EE. 1994. Apparently normal frequency of congenital anomalies in the highly polluted town of Cubatão, Brazil. *American Journal of Medical Genetics* 52(3):319–323.

Morrison G, Cronje AS, van Vuuren I, Op't Hof J. 1985. The incidence of cleft life and palate in the Western Cape. *South African Medical Journal* 68(8):576–577.

Murray JC, Daack-Hirsch S, Buetow KH, Munger R, Espina L, Paglinawan N, Villanueva E, Rary J, Magee K, Magee W. 1997. Clinical and epidemiologic studies of cleft lip and palate in the Philippines. *Cleft Palate-Craniofacial Journal* 34(1):7–10.

Murshid WR, Jarallah JS, Dad MI. 2000. Epidemiology of infantile hydrocephalus in Saudi Arabia: Birth prevalence and associated factors. *Pediatric Neurosurgery* 32(3):119–123.

Natsume N, Kawai T, Kohama G, Teshima T, Kochi S, Ohashi Y, Enomoto S, Ishii M, Nakano Y, Matsuya T, Kogo M, Yoshimura Y, Ohishi M, Nakamura N, Katsuki T, Goto M, Shimizu M, Yanagisawa S, Mimura T, Sunakawa H. 2000. Incidence of cleft lip or palate in 303,738 Japanese babies born between 1994 and 1995. *British Journal of Oral and Maxillofacial Surgery* 38(6):605–607.

Nazer HM. 1992. Early diagnosis of cystic fibrosis in Jordanian children. *Journal of Tropical Pediatrics* 38(3):113–115.

Niazi MA, al-Mazyad AS, al-Husain MA, al-Mofada SM, al-Zamil FA, Khashoggi TY, al-Eissa YA. 1995. Down's syndrome in Saudi Arabia: Incidence and cytogenetics. *Human Heredity* 45(2):65–69.

Nunes D, Dutra MG. 1986. Epidemiological study of congenital talipes calcaneovalgus. Brazilian Journal of Medical and Biological Research 19(1):59–62.

Ogle OE. 1993. Incidence of cleft lip and palate in a newborn Zairian sample. The Cleft Palate-Craniofacial Journal 30(2):250–251.

Op't Hof J, Venter PA, Louw M. 1991. Down's syndrome in South Africa: Incidence, maternal age and utilization of prenatal diagnosis. South African Medical Journal 79(4):213–216.

Ounap K, Lillevali H, Metspalu A, Lipping-Sitska M. 1998. Development of the phenylketonuria screening programme in Estonia. Journal of Medical Screening 5(1):22–23.

Ozalp I, Coskun T, Tokol S, Demircin G, Monch E. 1990. Inherited metabolic disorders in Turkey. Journal of Inherited Metabolic Disorders 13(5):732–738.

Padoa C, Goldman A, Jenkins T, Ramsay M. 1999. Cystic fibrois carrier frequencies in populations of African origin. Journal of Medical Genetics 36(1):41–44.

Peng GP, Chuan YT. 1988. Major congenital anomalies in livebirths in Alor Setar General Hospital during a three-year period. Medical Journal of Malaysia 43(2):138–149.

Pongpanich B, Dhanavaravibul S, Limsuwan A. 1976. Prevalence of heart disease in school children in Thailand: A preliminary survey at Bang Pa-in. Southeast Asian Journal of Tropical Medicine and Public Health 7(1):91–94.

Rajabian MH, Sherkat M. 2000. An epidemiologic study of oral clefts in Iran: Analysis of 1669 cases. The Cleft Palate-Craniofacial Journal 37(2):191–196.

Ramadevi R, Savithri HS, Devi AR, Bittles AH, Rao NA. 1994. An unusual distribution of glucose-6-phosphate dehydrogenase deficiency of south Indian newborn population. Indian Journal of Biochemistry and Biophysics 31(4):358–360.

Ramasamy S, Balakrishnan K, Pitchappan RM. 1994. Prevalence of sickle cells in Irula, Kurumba, Paniya and Mullukurumba tribes of Nilgiris (Tamil Nadu, India). Indian Journal of Medical Research 100:242–245.

Ratrisawadi V, Horpaopan S, Chotigeat U, Sangtawesin V, Kanjanapattanakul W, Ningsanond V, Sunthornthepvarakul T, Khooarmompatana S, Charoensiriwatana W. 1999. Neonatal screening program in Rajavithi Hospital, Thailand. Southeast Asian Journal of Tropical Medicine and Public Health 30(suppl 2):28–32.

Rawashdeh M, Manal H. 2000. Cystic fibrosis in Arabs: A prototype from Jordan. Annals of Tropical Pediatrics 20(4):283–286.

Reclos GJ, Hatzidakis CJ, Schulpis KH. 2000. Glucose-6-phosphate dehydrogenase deficiency neonatal screening: Preliminary evidence that a high percentage of partially deficient female neonates are missed during routine screening. Journal of Medical Screening 7(1):46–51.

Refat M, Rashad ES, El Gazar FA, Shafie AM, Abou El Nmour MM, Sherbini AE, El Soubky MK, Eissa AM. 1994. A clinicoepidemiologic study of heart disease in school children of Menoufia, Egypt. Annals of Saudi Medicine 14(3):225–229.

Rodríguez L, Sánchez R, Hernández J, Carrillo O, Heredero L. 1997. Results of 12 years' combined maternal serum alpha-fetoprotein screening and ultrasound fetal monitoring for prenatal detection of fetal malformations in Havana City, Cuba. Prenatal Diagnosis 17(4):301–304.

Salzano FM. 1985. Incidence, effects, and management of sickle cell disease in Brazil. American Journal of Pediatric Hematology/Oncology 7(3):240–244.

Sharma AK, Upreti M, Kamboj M, Mehra P, Das K, Misra A, Dhasmana S, Agarwal SS. 1994. Incidence of neural tube defects of Lucknow over a 10 year period from 1982–1991. Indian Journal of Medical Research 99:223–226.

Shi MN. 1989. Genetic epidemiological investigation of cleft lip and cleft palate [Article in Chinese]. Zhonghua Liu Xing Bing Xue Za Zhi 10(3):154–157.

Shija JK, Kingo ARM. 1985. A prospective clinical study of congenital anomalies seen at Harare Central Hospital, Zimbabwe. *Central African Journal of Medicine* 31(8):145–149.

Shohat M, Legum C, Romem Y, Borochowitz Z, Bach G, Goldman B. 1995. Down syndrome prevention program in a population with an older maternal age. *Obstetrics and Gynecology* (3):368–373.

Simpkiss M, Lowe A. 1961. Congenital abnormalities in the African newborn. *Archives of Disease in Childhood* 36:404–406.

Sin SY, Ghosh A, Tang LC, Chan V. 2000. Ten years' experience of antenatal mean corpuscular volume screening and prenatal diagnosis for thalassaemias in Hong Kong. *Journal of Obstetrics and Gynaecology Research* 26(3):203–208.

Singh H. 1986. Glucose-6-phosphate dehydrogenase deficiency: A preventable cause of mental retardation. *British Medical Journal* 292(6517):397–398.

Stout DB. 1942. San Blas acculturation. *Social Forces* 21:1.

Subramanyan R, Joy J, Venugopalan P, Sapru A, al Khusaiby SM. 2000. Incidence and spectrum of congenital heart disease in Oman. *Annals of Tropical Paediatrics* 20(4):337–341.

Sunna EI, Gharaibeh NS, Knapp DD, Bashir NA. 1996. Prevalence of hemoglobin S and beta-thalassemia in northern Jordan. *Journal of Obstetrics and Gynaecology Research* 22(1):17–20.

Talafih K, Hunaiti AA, Gharaibeh N, Gharaibeh M, Jaradat S. 1996. The prevalence of hemoglobin S and glucose-6-phosphate dehydrogenase deficiency in Jordanian newborn. *Journal of Obstetrics and Gynaecology Research* 22(5):417–420.

Tamagnini GP, Kuam B, Fai Wk. 1988. Congenital anemias in Macau. *Hemoglobin* 12(5–6):637–643.

Tan KI. 1988. Incidence and epidemiology of cleft lip/palate in Singapore. *Annals of the Academy of Medicine, Singapore* 17(3):311–314.

Tikkanen J, Heinonen OP. 1992. Occupational risk factors for congenital heart disease. *International Archives of Occupational and Environmental Health* 64(1):59–64.

Verma IC. 1978. High frequency of neural tube defects in North India. *Lancet* 1(8069):879–80.

Verma IC. 1986. Medical genetics in India. *Indian Journal of Pediatrics* 53(4):437–440.

Verma IC. 1988. Genetics causes of mental retardation. In Niermeijer M, Hicks E (eds.). *Mental Retardation, Genetics and Ethical Considerations*. Amsterdam: Reidel Publishing Co. Pp. 99–106.

Verma IC, Elango R, Mehta L. 1990. Monitoring reproductive and developmental effects of environmental factors in India: A review. In *All India Institute of Medical Sciences*. Pp. 63–73.

Verma IC, Anand NK, Modi UJ, Bharucha BA. 1998. *Study of Malformations and Down Syndrome in India: A Multicentric Study*. Trombay, Mumbai: Department of Atomic Energy, Bhabha Atomic Research Center.

Venter PA, Christianson AL, Hutamo CM, Makhura MP, Gericke GS. 1995. Congenital anomalies in rural black South African neonates: A silent epidemic? *South African Medical Journal* 85(1):15–20.

Wu Y, Zeng M, Xu C, Liang J, Wang Y, Miao L, Xiao K. 1995. Analyses of the prevalences for neural tube defects and cleft lip and palate in China from 1988 to 1991. *Hua Xi Yi Ke Da Xue Xue Bao* 26(2):215–219.

Wurie AT, Wurie IM, Gevao SM, Robbin-Coker DJ. 1996. The prevalence of sickle cell trait in Sierra Leone. A laboratory profile. *West African Journal of Medicine* 15(4):201–203.

Xiao GZ, Zhang ZY, Li JC, et al. 1989. Epidemic investigation of cleft lip and palate in China [Article in Chinese]. *Chinese Medical Journal* 69:192.

Xiao KZ, Zhang ZY, Su YM, Liu FQ, Yan ZZ, Jiang ZQ, Zhou SF, He WG, Wang BY, Jiang HP. 1990. Central nervous system congenital malformations, especially neural tube defects in 29 provinces, metropolitan cities and autonomous regions of China: Chinese Birth Defects Monitoring Program. *International Journal of Epidemiology* 19(4):978–982.

Zhang Z, Li Z, Ji C. 1990. Prevalence study of congenital heart disease in children aged 0–2 in Zhejiang Province [Article in Chinese]. *Zhonghua Liu Xing Bing Xue Za Zhi* 20(3):155–157.

Appendix B

Committee Biographies

ADETOKUNBO O. LUCAS, M.D. (Co-chair), was born in Nigeria and obtained his medical degree at Durham University, England. His postgraduate training in internal medicine, public health, and tropical medicine took him to Belfast, London, and Harvard University. He chaired the Department for Preventive and Social Medicine in Ibaden, Nigeria, until 1976. From 1976 to 1986, he directed the Tropical Diseases Research Programme of the World Health Organization, and from 1986 to 1990, he served as the chair of the Carnegie Corporation's Strengthening Human Resources in Developing Countries grant program. In 1990, Dr. Lucas was appointed professor of international health at the Harvard School of Public Health. He has served on the technical advisory boards of several national organizations and international agencies including the Rockefeller Foundation, the Edna McConnell Clark Foundation, the Carter Center, and the Welcome Trust Scientific Group on Tropical Medicine. He now chairs the Global Forum for Health Research. Dr. Lucas has received academic honors from Harvard University and honorary degrees from Emory, Tulane, and Ibadan Universities. He is a fellow of the Royal College of Obstetricians and Gynaecologists and is one of the first foreign associates of the Institute of Medicine.

BARBARA J. STOLL, M.D. (Co-chair), received her medical degree from Yale Medical School, completed a pediatric residency at Babies Hospital, Columbia Presbyterian Medical Center, and a neonatology fellowship at Emory University School of Medicine. She is currently professor of pediatrics at Emory and vice-chair for research in the Department of Pediatrics. She spent four years working on issues of childhood disease and mortality at the International Center for Diarrhoeal Disease Research, Bangladesh. In 1995–1996 she was a visiting scientist at the World Health Organization. She is currently a member of the Advisory Board for the Saving Newborn Lives Initiative of Save the Children, a member of the Society for Pediatric Research, the Perinatal Research Society, the American Pediatric Society, and a fellow of the American Academy of Pediatrics and the Infectious Diseases Society of America. Her extensive research and publications have focused on low birth weight and premature newborns, preventing and treating neonatal infections, and the global impact of neonatal infections. Dr. Stoll is on the Steering Committee of the National Institute of Child Health and Human Development Neonatal Research Network and is one of the principal investigators of the collaborative network. In addition, Dr. Stoll practices neonatology at Emory University in Atlanta, Georgia.

ANNA ALISJAHBANA, M.D., Ph.D., is professor emeritus of pediatrics in the School of Medicine at Padjadjaran University in Indonesia and Director of the World Health Organization Collaborating Center for Perinatal and Maternal and Child Care in Indonesia. She has studied many aspects of perinatal care, including community-based training of traditional birth attendants in rural areas. In addition, Dr. Alisjahbana has served as a technical consultant for the Asian Development Bank, World Health Organization, United Nations Children's Fund, and the government of Indonesia on a number of programs to improve perinatal outcomes and early child development. She has published on a range topics including patterns of birthweight in rural Indonesia, prevention of hypothermia in low weight infants, ways to improve health care services to prevent maternal mortality, and appropriate technology for resuscitation of newborns. She is founder and chairperson of Surya Kanti Foundation, a nonprofit organization working with children 0–5 years of age with developmental disabilities. The foundation clinic provides services to more than 8,000 patients per year.

ABHAY BANG, M.D., M.P.H., received his M.P.H. from Johns Hopkins School of Public Health. He is currently living, working, and conducting research in Gadchiroli, India, where he is the director of the Society for Education, Action, and Research in Community Health. After establishing baseline data on birth outcomes in the Maharastra region of India, Dr. Bang is studying the efficacy of pairing trained village birth attendants with traditional birth attendants in rural settings in India. As a pediatrician, working in tandem with his wife, an obstetrician, he is providing care, training village birth workers, and monitoring the data on improved birth outcomes.

LAURA CAULFIELD, Ph.D., received her doctorate in international nutrition from Cornell University. In 1990, she joined the faculty of the Johns Hopkins School of Public Health and is currently associate professor in the Division of Human Nutrition, Department of International Health. Dr. Caulfield has studied the role of nutrition in improving birth outcomes in diverse populations, including the United States and Canada, Latin America, and South Asia. Currently, she is conducting research on the role of prenatal iron and zinc supplements for improving infant health in Peru. Dr. Caulfield has served as a consultant to the Pan American Health Organization, the United States Agency for International Development, and numerous private voluntary organizations. She is a member of various societies, including the Society for International Nutrition Research and the Society for Pediatric and Perinatal Epidemiologic Research, and is vice-chair of the Nutritional Epidemiology Research Interest Section of the American Society of Nutritional Sciences.

ROBERT GOLDENBERG, M.D., received his medical training from Duke University. He is professor of public health and Charles E. Flowers Professor and Chair of the Department of Obstetrics and Gynecology at the University of Alabama, Birmingham, where he also served as the irector of the Center for Obstetric Research for 10 years. He currently directs the Center for Research in Women's Health. Dr. Goldenberg was director of obstetrical services at Cooper Green Hospital in Birmingham from 1986 to 1989 and chairman of the Department of Obstetrics and Gynecology at Cooper Green Hospital from 1987 to 1991. He is a member of the Institute of Medicine and chairman of the Membership Committee for Pediatrics, and Obstetrics and Gynecology. He has served on numerous advisory committees, including the Council for the National Institute of Child Health and Human Development; the National Institutes of Health Expert Panels on the Content of Prenatal Care and on Pregnancy, Birth, and the Infant Research Plan; and the Congressional Office of Technology Assessment Child Health Advisory Panel. Dr. Goldenberg has been the principal investigator on major grants from the National Institute of Child Health and Human Development, the National Institute of Allergy and Infectious Diseases, the March of Dimes, and the Robert Wood Johnson Foundation. He has published extensively on preterm birth prediction, low birth weight, intrauterine growth retardation, neonatal mortality, and maternal and neonatal infectious disease prevention, diagnosis, and treatment.

MARJORIE KOBLINSKY, Ph.D., received her doctorate in biochemistry from Columbia University and also holds a certificate of community medicine and health from the Liverpool School of Tropical Medicine. Dr. Koblinsky is project director of MotherCare at the John Snow, Inc., Center for Women's Health where she is responsible for multiple projects aimed at developing, implementing, and evaluating a community-based approach to improving maternal and neonatal health and nutrition in developing countries, including Indonesia, India, Pakistan, Nigeria, Uganda, Kenya, Zambia, Bolivia, Ecuador, Peru, and Guatemala. She has also been a program officer for the Ford Foundation and the Canadian International Development Research Center and a project director and research scientist at the International Center for Diarrhoeal Disease Research in Bangladesh. Dr. Koblinsky has published on a range of topics related to maternal health and survival, including ways to define and measure maternal mortality and morbidity, methods for achieving healthy pregnancies and safe deliveries, and implementing and evaluating programs in reproductive health and family planning. She is the 1993 recipient of the National Council for International Health (NCIH) International Health Award, and her project, Mother- Care, was the 1998 recipient of the World Health Day Award, given by the American Association of World Health.

MICHAEL KRAMER, M.D., received his M.D., pediatrics, and epidemiology training at the Yale University School of Medicine. Since 1978, he has been at the McGill University Faculty of Medicine and, since 1987, he has been a professor in the Departments of Pediatrics and of Epidemiology and Biostatistics. He is currently a distinguished scientist of the Medical Research Council of Canada. His research focuses on perinatal epidemiology and currently includes a multicenter randomized trial of the World Health Organization/United Nations Children's Fund Baby-Friendly Hospital Initiative to promote breastfeeding; development of new fetal growth standards based on early ultrasound-validated gestational age; international comparisons of fetal and infant mortality; and mechanisms and causal pathways underlying socioeconomic disparities in risk for preterm birth.

AFFETTE McCAW-BINNS, Ph.D., received her doctorate in perinatal epidemiology from the University of Bristol in England. She is a lecturer in the Department of Community Health and Psychiatry at the University of the West Indies, Mona, in Kingston, Jamaica, and a visiting lecturer at the University of Connecticut School of Public Health. Her research is concerned with the epidemiology of perinatal deaths and maternal mortality in the Caribbean, as well as antenatal and perinatal care in that region. She has recently published *Informing Maternal and Child Health Policy Through Research*. Dr. McCaw-Binns is a member of the Pan American Health Organization's Technical and Advisory Group of the Regional Plan for Action for the Reduction of Maternal Mortality in the Americas.

KUSUM J. NATHOO, M.B., Ch.B., M.R.C.P., D.C.H., is associate professor of pediatrics and child health in the Medical School and member of the Clinical Epidemiology Unit at the University of Zimbabwe in Harare. She has studied the effects of several infectious diseases on maternal and infant survival. Her research has addressed many topics ranging from the transmission of HIV from mother to infant and mortality within the first two years among infants born to HIV-infected women, to predictors of mortality in children hospitalized with diseases such as dysentery, bacteremia, measles, and bronchopneumonia. Dr. Nathoo has contributed significantly through her research to the understanding of trends in child health and survival in Zimbabwe and in Africa.

HARSHADKUMAR CHANDULAL SANGHVI, M.B., Ch.B., has more than 15 years of experience in Africa as a clinical service provider and university faculty and researcher in obstetrics and gynecology. In his current position as the medical director of the Maternal and Neonatal Program at the Johns Hopkins Program for International Education in Gynecology and Obstetrics in Baltimore Maryland, he is responsible for the development of reproductive health training materials, especially those for maternal and neonatal health care. He is a senior associate at the School of Public Health, Johns Hopkins University. As the chair of his department at the University of Nairobi in Kenya, he played an instrumental role in the promotion of preservice training for medical students and postgraduates in all aspects of reproductive care. He has been involved in designing and implementing large-scale epidemiological studies including the Nairobi Birth Survey and the four-country East Central and Southern African Maternal Mortality Study. His many publications include studies on adolescent health, family planning, maternal and neonatal health, and cervical cancer.

JOE LEIGH SIMPSON, M.D., received his medical education and training at Duke University and Cornell Medical College. Dr. Simpson is Ernst W. Bertner Chairman and Professor of Obstetrics & Gynecology and professor of molecular and human genetics at Baylor College of Medicine in Houston. His investigative pursuits center on reproductive genetics: prenatal genetic diagnosis and preimplantation genetics, genetics of spontaneous abortion, elucidation of disorders of sexual differentiation, and determination of the causes of chromosomal nondisjunction. Dr. Simpson was 1993–1994 president of the American Society for Reproductive Medicine, 1994–1998 president of the International Society of Prenatal Diagnosis, 1995–1998 president of the Society for Advancement of Contraception, and 1998–1999 president of the Society for Gynecologic Investigation. He is a member of the March of Dimes Scientific Advisory Board and was a member from 1995 to 1997 of the National Institute of Child Health and

Human Development Advisory Council. In 1995 he was elected to the Institute of Medicine. He is treasurer or the American College of Medical Genetics and has assumed many responsibilities for the American College of Obstetricians and Gynecologists. He has published extensively in the fields of obstetrics and gynecology, clinical genetics, and etiology of birth defects. Dr. Simpson has received major research funding from the March of Dimes, the National Institutes of Health, and the U.S. Agency for International Development.

Glossary

Alpha-fetoprotein blood test: A test performed on a pregnant women to identify the presence of a particular protein, which suggests that the fetus has a neural tube defect.

Amniocentesis: The sampling of the fluid surrounding the fetus to provide a test for specific conditions such as Down syndrome or spina bifida.

Amniotic fluid: The fluid that, contained in the sac of membranes known as the amnion, surrounds the fetus and provides a shock absorber and a secondary vehicle for the exchange of body chemicals with the mother.

Anemia: The condition of having fewer than the normal number of red blood cells, or hemoglobin, in the blood, which causes patients to fatigue easily, appear pale, develop palpitations, and become short of breath. There are many causes of anemia, including bleeding, abnormal hemoglobin formation (such as in sickle cell anemia), iron, B_{12} (pernicious anemia), or folic acid deficiency, rupture of red blood cells (hemolytic anemia), and bone marrow diseases.

Anencephaly: Congenital absence of the cranial vault with cerebral hemispheres missing or reduced to small masses attached to the base of the skull.

Antenatal: Before birth; also called prenatal.

Autosomal disorder: If a disorder is autosomal it is found on both the X and Y chromosomes. (Each child receives one chromosome from each parent. The mother has 2 X chromosomes so always gives a X. The father has an X and a Y: when he gives an X, it is a female child, and when he gives a Y, it is a male child).

Behavioral change: A change in habits or lifestyle that can be characterized as proceeding through four stages: precontemplation, contemplation, action, and maintenance of a new behavior.

Bilirubin: A breakdown product of heme that normally circulates in plasma as a complex with albumin. It is taken up by the liver and conjugated to form bilirubin diglucuronide, which is excreted in bile. Unconjugated bilirubin is not excreted in the urine, which can lead to an excess of bilirubin in the blood (jaundice).

Birth defect: Any structural or functional abnormality determined by factors operating largely before conception or during gestation.

Birth defects of complex and unknown origin: Birth defects with unknown origins and likely to be due to the additive effects of a few or many genes, which may interact with nongenetic or environmental factors.

Birth prevalence: The number of individuals who have an attribute or disease at the time of birth divided by the population at risk of having the attribute or disease the time of birth.

Capacity building: Increasing the ability of a local institution to provide high-quality services appropriate to the local setting, which involves performance assessment and targeted strategies to improve staff competency, logistics, and other determinants of quality of care.

Carrier: One who carries and may transmit a genetic defect or infectious agent in the absence of symptoms.

Chorionic villus sampling: A procedure in which a small sample of cells is removed from the placenta where it joins the uterus. The cells are used to test for chromosomal abnormalities in the fetus, such as Down syndrome.

Chromosomal disorders: Sporadic nonhereditary losses or rearrangements of genetic material.

Chromosomal nondisjunction: An error in cell division that admits three, rather than two, copies of one of the chromosomes into the cells of the affected zygote. Three copies (trisomy) of chromosome 21 cause Down syndrome.

Cleft lip and/or palate: A gap in the soft palate and roof of the mouth, sometimes extending through the upper lip. This condition occurs when the various parts of a lip or palate don't grow together to make a single lip or hard palate. It is usually correctable. Eating, speech production, hearing, and tooth formation are all affected by this condition.

Clinical trial: A scientifically controlled study carried out in people with a particular disease or class of diseases to test the effectiveness of a treatment or a method of prevention, detection, or diagnosis.

Community-based rehabilitation (CBR): A strategy in communities for the rehabilitation, equalization of opportunities, and social integration of people with disabilities. The strategy mobilizes local resources and enables people with disabilities and their communities to create their own solutions and programs for rehabilitation.

Congenital abnormality: An anomaly, deformity, malformation, impairment, or dysfunction that is present at birth, but not necessarily inherited.

Congenital cytomegalovirus: Fetal infection with cytomegalovirus causes disease only in utero, but this can result in abortion, stillbirth, or various congenital defects. Persons who have been exposed to the virus will remain cytomegalovirus IgG-positive. Infected cells enlarge and have a characteristic inclusion body (composed of virus particles) in the nucleus.

Congenital heart disease: A malformation of the heart or large blood vessels near the heart that is present at birth. This is the most common of the major birth defects and affects 8 per 1,000 live births.

Congenital hypothyroidism: Lack of thyroid secretion due to inappropriate development of the thymus gland or inadequate maternal iodine intake during gestation which leads to stunted body growth and mental development in the first years of life.

Congenital rubella syndrome: Fetal infection with rubella virus during the first trimester of pregnancy can cause a series of congenital abnormalities including heart disease, deafness, and blindness.

Congenital: A condition or disease that is present at birth. It includes conditions that are inherited and others caused by a new genetic mutation or an environmental exposure.

Consanguineous: Related by blood. Consanguineous marriage usually refers to the marriage of first cousins but includes second cousins.

Convulsion: A sudden attack usually characterized by loss of consciousness and sustained or rhythmic contractions of some or all voluntary muscles. Convulsions are most often a manifestation of a seizure disorder (epilepsy).

Cost-effectiveness analysis: A systematic methodology for the comparison of the overall costs and health benefits of public health interventions.

Cretinism: Congenital hypothyroidism (underactivity of the thyroid gland at birth) resulting in growth retardation, developmental delay, and other abnormal features. Can be due to deficiency of iodine in the mother's diet during pregnancy or inappropriate development of the thymus gland.

Cyanosis: The bluish color of the skin and mucous membranes due to insufficient oxygen in the blood.

Cystic fibrosis (CF): A generalized disorder in which there is widespread dysfunction of the exocrine glands, characterized by signs of chronic pulmonary disease (due to excess mucus production in the respiratory tract), pancreatic deficiency, abnormally high levels of electrolytes in the sweat, and occasionally by biliary cirrhosis. There is an ineffective immunological defense against bacteria in the lungs. Without treatment, CF results in death for 95 percent of affected children before age five. With diligent medical care patients with CF can survive beyond middle age.

Developing countries: Defined by the World Bank as countries with per capita income below $2996 in 2001. Low-income countries had a per capita income of $755 or less in 2001. Middle-income countries had a per capita income of $756–$2,995 in 2001.

Developmental dysplasia of the hip (DDH): DDH is a malformation of the hip joint in which the head of the femur is not correctly positioned in the acetabulum. The cause is unknown, but genetic factors may play a role. Problems range from congenital dislocation of the hip where the head of the femur is completely outside the acetabulum and the hip is very unstable to conditions where the displacement shortens one leg and causes limping, joint and knee problems, and degenerative changes.

Diagnosis: Identification of a disease or disorder.

Disability-adjusted life years (DALY): An indicator that combines losses from premature death (the difference between the actual age at death and life expectancy in a low-mortality population) and loss of healthy life resulting from disability.

Dominant: A mode of inheritance in which the gene from one parent is required for a trait to appear in an offspring.

Down syndrome: A common chromosomal disorder in which a person is born with three—not two—copies of chromosome number 21 (trisomy 21). It causes mental retardation, a characteristic facial appearance, and multiple malformations. It is associated with a major risk for heart malformations, a risk of duodenal atresia in which part of the small intestine is not developed, and a small but significant risk of acute leukemia. Down syndrome can be detected in the first few months of pregnancy by amniocentesis. The risk factors include mothers who become pregnant after age 35 and having a prior child with Down syndrome. This disorder was formerly known as mongolism.

Effective treatment: The effect of a treatment as observed in the controlled circumstances of a clinical trial.

Efficacious treatment: The effect of a treatment that can be expected in real clinical practice.

Encephalocele: A protrusion of the brain or part of the brain through a fissure in the bones of the skull.

Environmental birth defect: A defect present in a baby at birth, caused by prenatal events that are not genetic. These include maternal infections, certain medications, some drugs, and ionizing radiation.

Evidence-based medicine/health care: In evidence-based health care, the policies and practices used for prevention are based on principles that have been proven through appropriate scientific methods. As well as proving the clinical effectiveness of a procedure, this involves evidence of user and provider satisfaction, feasibility, and cost-effectiveness of the procedure in different settings.

Fetal alcohol syndrome: A clinical syndrome resulting from the direct toxic effects of alcohol on the developing fetus. Growth retardation, mental retardation, small brain, and heart valve lesions are common. Infants can be identified by close-set eyes, small head, small nasal bridge, reduction in the vermilion border of the upper lip, eye folds, and small teeth.

Genetic birth defect: A defect present in a baby at birth, caused by a genetic factor.

Genetic screening test: A test that identifies clinically normal individuals who have genotypes associated with a birth defect or who are at high risk of producing offspring with a birth defect. Genetic screening of large populations aims to identify as many affected individuals as possible, but screening alone does not detect all individuals at high risk.

Gestational age: The number of completed weeks since the last menstrual period of the mother. This can be assessed clinically or by obstetric ultrasound.

Glucose-6-phosphate dehydrogenase (G6PD) deficiency: This enzyme defect occurs on the X chromosome. Males with the enzyme deficiency develop anemia due to breakup of their red blood cells when they are exposed to oxidant drugs such as the antimalarial, primaquine, the sulfonamide antibiotics or sulfones, naphthalene mothballs, or fava beans. Fever, viral and bacterial infections, and diabetic acidosis can also precipitate a hemolytic crisis (when the red blood cells break up), resulting in anemia and jaundice. This is the commonest disease-causing enzyme defect in humans, affecting an estimated 400 million people. It occurs with increased frequency in people of sub-Saharan African or Mediterranean origin. The concentration of G6PD deficiency in certain populations is the result of the protective effect it afforded (much like sickle cell trait) against malaria.

Goiter: Enlargement of the thyroid gland. Goiter can be associated with levels of thyroid hormone that are normal, too high, or too low.

Hemizygote: Nucleus, cell, or organism that has only one of a normally diploid set of genes. In mammals the male is hemizygous for the X chromosome.

Hemolysis: The destruction of red blood cells, which leads to the release of hemoglobin into the blood plasma.

Hemolytic jaundice: Jaundice (yellowing) caused by destruction of red blood cells. This can be an inborn condition (hereditary spherocytosis) or it may be caused by a blood transfusion from a different blood group, infection in the blood, or some types of poisoning.

Hemophilia A and B: A hemorrhagic diathesis occurring in two main forms, both determined by a mutant gene of the X chromosome. The disease is characterized by subcutaneous and intramuscular hemorrhages; bleeding from the mouth, gums, lips, and tongue; hematuria; and hemarthroses. Hemophilia A (classic hemophilia, factor VIII deficiency) is an X-linked disorder due to deficiency of coagulation factor VIII, and hemophilia B (factor IX deficiency, Christmas disease), also X linked, is due to deficiency of coagulation factor IX.

Hepatomegaly: Enlargement of the liver.

Hereditary: Refers to a disease or condition that is passed from parents to child.

Heterozygote: Nucleus, cell, or organism with different alleles of one or more specific genes. A heterozygous organism will produce unlike gametes and thus will not breed true.

Holoprosencephaly: A disorder characterized by the failure of the embryonic forebrain to divide to form bilateral cerebral hemispheres (the left and right halves of the brain), causing defects in the development of the face and in brain structure and function.

Homozygote: Nucleus, cell, or organism with identical alleles of one or more specific genes; a person who has two identical forms of a particular gene, one inherited from each parent.

Hydranencephaly: A condition in which the cerebral hemispheres of the brain are absent and replaced by sacs filled with cerebrospinal fluid. The cerebellum and brainstem are usually formed normally.

Hydrocephalus: Hydrocephalus is an abnormal buildup of cerebrospinal fluid (CSF) in the ventricles of the brain. The fluid is often under increased pressure and can compress and damage the brain.

Hyperbilirubinemia: An excess of bilirubin in the blood.

Hyperthermia: Abnormally high body temperature.

Immune: Protected against infection.

In utero: Within the womb. .

Incidence: The number of new cases of a disease among a certain group of people for a certain period of time.

Infant mortality rate (IMR): Number of deaths among infants under one year of age per 1,000 live births.

Infarction: The formation of an area of tissue death because of a local lack of oxygen.

Insulin-dependent diabetes mellitus (IDDM): A chronic condition in which the pancreas makes little or no insulin because the beta cells have been destroyed. Insulin is required for the breakdown of glucose (blood sugar) for energy. IDDM usually occurs abruptly, although the damage to the beta cells may begin much earlier. The signs of IDDM are a great thirst, hunger, a need to urinate often, and loss of weight. Treatment of the disease involves insulin injections, a specific diet plan, daily exercise, and frequent testing of blood glucose levels. IDDM usually occurs in children and adults under the age of 30. This type of diabetes used to be known as juvenile diabetes, juvenile-onset diabetes, and ketosis-prone diabetes.

Intracranial calcification: The process within the skull by which organic tissue becomes hardened by a deposit of calcium salts within its substance.

Iodine deficiency disorder: Iodine is a dietary requirement, and inadequate intake causes inadequate production of thyroid hormone (hypothyroidism).

Ischemia: A low oxygen state usually due to obstruction of the arterial blood supply or inadequate blood flow leading to hypoxia in the tissue.

Jaundice: A condition in which high levels of bilirubin in the blood cause a yellow coloration in the skin.

Kernicterus: Disorder in a newborn baby caused by high levels of bilirubin in the blood. When bilirubin is deposited in the brain it causes bilirubin encephalopathy.

Live birth: A baby born with any signs of life, independently of weight or gestation.

Low birth weight (LBW): Birth weight less than 2,500 grams.

Macrosomia: Larger-than-normal birth weight, usually more than 9.75 pounds, or 4,500 grams.

Management: A process by which one plans, implements, and evaluates an organized response to a health problem.

Meningoencephalitis: Inflammation of both the brain and meninges, which are the membranes surrounding the brain and spinal cord.

Meta-analysis: The statistical method used to integrate results from more than one study to produce a summary estimate of the treatment effect across studies (typical relative risk).

Morbidity: Departure from a state of physiological or psychological well-being.

Multiple gestation: More than one fetus developing in the uterus.

Mutation: A change in genetic material that occurs by chance.

Myelomeningocele: The protrusion of the spinal cord and its membranes.

Myxedema: A dry, waxy type of swelling, often with swollen lips and nose, which results from infantile hypothyroidism.

Neonate: An infant in the time between birth and 28 completed days of life (the neonatal period).

Neural tube defects (NTDs): Major birth defects caused by abnormal development of the neural tube, the structure present during embryonic life that gives rise to the central nervous system, brain, and spinal cord. Neural tube defects (NTDs) are among the most common birth defects that cause death and serious disability. The different types of NTDs include anencephaly, spina bifida, and encephalocele.

Neural tube: A structure in early fetal life that develops into the brain, spinal cord, spinal nerves, and spine.

Non-consanguineous: Not related by blood—referring to the parents of an offspring.

Nystagmus: An involuntary, rapid, rhythmic movement of the eyeball, which may be horizontal, vertical, rotatory, or mixed.

Obstructed labor: Labor in which progress is arrested by mechanical factors. Delivery may require cesarean section.

Occiput: The back of the head.

Oculocutaneous albinism: An autosomal recessive deficiency of pigment in skin, hair, and eyes; in the tyrosinase-negative type, there is an absence of tyrosinase; in the tyrosinase-positive type, the normal tyrosinase cannot enter pigment cells. There are several types of oculocutaneous albinism.

Parity: Number of full-term children previously born by a woman, excluding miscarriages and abortions in early pregnancy, but including stillbirths.

Phenylketonuria: Congenital absence of phenylalanine hydroxylase (the enzyme that converts phenylalanine to tyrosine). Phenylalanine accumulates in blood and seriously impairs early neuronal development.

Photophobia: Painful oversensitivity to light.

Polydactyly: More than the normal number of fingers or toes.

Prenatal: The period of time between the conception and birth of an infant. Also called antenatal.

Prevalence: The number of instances of a given disease or other condition in a particular population at a specified time.

Pulmonary hypertension: High blood pressure in the pulmonary arteries, which can irrevocably damage the lungs.

Randomized controlled trials (RCT): Trial experiments in which investigators randomly allocate eligible people or health care units into groups to receive, or not receive, the intervention(s) being compared. When sample size is adequate, randomization ensures baseline comparability of known and unknown prognostic variables. The outcomes are selected before the experiment to ensure an unbiased assessment of the results.

Recessive: A mode of inheritance in which a gene must be present from both parents for the trait to become manifest in an offspring.

Reduction deformities of limbs: Congenital absence or attenuation of one or more body parts.

Relative risk: The ratio of the risk of death or disease in those exposed to the risk compared with the risk in those not exposed.

Seizure: A sudden attack of epileptic convulsion in which the patient may experience uncontrollable body movements, unusual smells or tastes, or loss of consciousness.

Sickle cell disease: Also known as sickle cell anemia, this is a genetic blood disease that results from the pairing of an abnormal hemoglobin S (Hb S) with another abnormal hemoglobin; the most frequent and severe phenotypes are hemoglobin SS (Hb SS) and hemoglobin SC (Hb SC). The hemoglobin molecules in red blood cells stick to one another and cause the red cells to become crescent- or sickle-shaped. Sickled cells cannot pass easily through tiny blood vessels. Sickle cell disease affects millions of people worldwide but is particularly common among people from sub-Saharan Africa; Spanish-speaking regions; Saudi Arabia; India; and Mediterranean countries.

Spina bifida: Incomplete closure of the spinal cord through which the cord and meninges may or may not protrude.

Splenomegaly: Enlargement of the spleen.

Spontaneous abortion: A pregnancy in which the fetus cannot survive or in which the fetus is born before the 20th week of pregnancy. Also known as a miscarriage.

Squamous cell carcinoma: Cancer that begins in squamous cells, which are found in the tissue that forms the surface of the skin, the lining of the hollow organs of the body, and the passages of the respiratory and digestive tracts.

Stillbirth: The death of a fetus weighing at least 500 g (or when birth weight is unavailable, after 22 completed weeks of gestation or with a crown-heel length of 25 cm or more), before the complete expulsion or extraction from its mother.

Stillborn infant: An infant who shows no evidence of life after birth.

Surveillance: The systematic collection and analysis of data in order to make management decisions.

Syncope: Partial or complete loss of consciousness with a spontaneous recovery.

Talipes, or clubfoot: This is the most common congenital abnormality of the foot. It may occur in several forms. Talipes equinovarus is the most common and in this case the foot turns downward and inward. Treatment involves the extended use of orthopedic splints or casts to correct the position of the foot.

Talocalcaneonavicular (joint): A ball-and-socket synovial joint, part of which participates in the transverse tarsal joint, formed by the head of the talus articulating with the navicular bone and the anterior part of the calcaneus.

Teratogen: Any agent that can disturb the development of an embryo or fetus, which may halt the pregnancy or cause a birth defect in the child. Teratogens include some maternal infections, chemicals, drugs, and radiation.

Thalassemias: These are a group of inherited blood disorders in which production of hemoglobin is deficient. There are many different disorders involving defective hemoglobin synthesis and, hence, many types of thalassemia.

- α-Thalassemia, the heterozygous state (with a single gene for alphathalassemia) is innocuous or harmless. The homozygous state (with both genes for alpha-thalassemia) can be lethal before birth.
- β-Thalassemia involves a defect in the production of beta-globin chains, which decreases production of normal adult hemoglobin (Hb A), the predominant type of hemoglobin from soon after birth until death. This is the most common thalassemia.

Therapeutic: Pertaining to treatment.

Total births: All births, live and stillborn (late fetal deaths).

Toxoplasmosis: An acute or chronic widespread disease caused by the protozoan *Toxoplasma gondii* and transmitted by oocysts containing the pathogen in the feces of cats (the definitive host), contaminated soil, direct exposure to infected feces, tissue cysts in infected meat or tachyzoites (proliferating forms) in blood.

Trisomy 13 syndrome: Children with this syndrome have three, instead of two, copies of chromosome 13. Children born with this syndrome have multiple malformations and mental retardation, including scalp defects, blood vessel malformations of the face and nape of the neck, cleft lip and palate, malformations of the heart and abdominal organs, and flexed fingers with extra digits. The mental retardation is profound, with an IQ that is too low to accurately test. The majority of trisomy 13 babies die soon after birth or in infancy. The condition is also called Patau syndrome.

Trisomy 18 syndrome: Children with this syndrome have three, instead of two, copies of chromosome 18. This condition causes multiple malformations and profound mental retardation, small head (microcephaly), small jaw (micrognathia), malformations of the heart and kidneys, clenched fists with abnormal finger positioning, malformed feet, and low birth weight. The vast majority (95 percent) of these children die before their first birthday. The condition is also called Edwards syndrome.

Ultrasound: A diagnostic procedure that projects high-frequency sound waves into the body and converts the echoes into pictures (sonograms) shown on a monitor. Different types of tissue reflect sound waves differently, which makes it possible to find abnormal growths.

Ultraviolet radiation: Invisible rays of solar energy. Ultraviolet radiation can burn the skin and cause skin cancer. It is made up of two types of rays, UVA and UVB. UVB rays are more likely than UVA rays to cause sunburn, but UVA rays pass further into the skin. Scientists have long thought that UVB radiation can cause melanoma and other types of skin cancer. UVA radiation is now considered to add skin damage that can lead to cancer. Sunscreens are recommended to block both kinds of radiation.

Vital registration: Identifying and recording every birth and death of a pregnant woman and newborn.

X-linked: A disorder found only on the X chromosome. If a male child (XY) has an X-linked disorder, it was passed on by the mother. If a female child (XX) has an X-linked disorder, the defective gene could have come from either parent.

Definitions for this glossary were compiled from the following sources:

Birth Disorder Information Directory. Available at http://www.bdid.com/.

MedicineNet, Inc. *MedTerms Medical Dictionary.* Available at http://www. MedicineNet.com, 2003.

MedlinePlus. The National Library of Medicine (date of last update: 21 November 2002). Available at http://www.nlm.nih.gov/medlineplus/.

CancerWEB. The Department of Medical Oncology at the University of Newcastle upon Tyne. Available at http://cancerweb.ncl.ac.uk/omd/index.html, 2003.

Acronyms

ARND	alcohol-related neurodevelopmental disorder
BPF	Bangladesh Protibondhi Foundation
CARE	Cooperative for Assistance and Relief Everywhere
CBDMP	Chinese Birth Defects Monitoring Program
CBR	community-based rehabilitation
CEUs	clinical epidemiology units
CF	cystic fibrosis
CHD	congenital heart disease
CID	generalized cytomegalic inclusion disease
CMV	congenital cytomegalovirus
CNS	central nervous system
CRS	congenital rubella syndrome
CRU	children's rehabilitation unit
CVS	chorionic villus sampling
DALY	disability-adjusted life years
DDH	developmental dysplasia of the hip
DNA	deoxyribonucleic acid
ECLAMC	Latin American Collaborative Study of Congenital Malformations
ELISA	enzyme-linked immunosorbent assay
EUROCAT	European Register of Congenital Abnormalities and Twins
FAS	fetal alcohol syndrome
G6PD	glucose-6-phosphate dehydrogenase
Hb	hemoglobin

HbS	sickle cell hemoglobin
HbSC	hemoglobin C
HbSE	hemoglobin E
HbSS	sickle cell anemia
hCG	human chorionic gonadotropin
HIV/AIDS	human immunodeficiency virus/acquired immune deficiency syndrome
HSV	herpes simplex virus
HSV-1	herpes simplex virus type 1
HSV-2	herpes simplex virus type 2
ICBDMS	International Clearinghouse for Birth Defects Monitoring System
IDDM	insulin-dependent diabetes mellitus
IDDs	iodine deficiency disorders
IEF	isoelectric focusing
IgM	immunoglobulin M
INCLEN	International Clinical Epidemiology Network
IOM	Institute of Medicine
IQ	intelligence quotient
KFMI	Korean Federation of Medical Insurance
MCH	maternal and child health
MMR	measles-mumps-rubella
NGOs	nongovernmental organizations
NTD	neural tube defect
O-B	Ortolani-Barlow
PATH	Program for Appropriate Technology in Health
PCR	polymerase chain reaction
PDA	patent ductus arteriosus
PKU	phenylketonuria
PS	pulmonary stenosis
RA 27/3	rubella vaccine
RBC	red blood cel
SCD	sickle cell disease
SPF	sun protection factor
STDs	sexually transmitted diseases
STI	sexually transmitted infections
TDR	Research and Training in Tropical Diseases
UNESCO	United Nations Educational, Scientific and Cultural Organization
VSD	ventricular septal defect
WHO	World Health Organization

Index

A

Abortion
  counseling, 106
  ethical issues, 108
  induced or spontaneous, 2, 4, 5, 8, 23,
      25, 26, 45, 52, 84, 98, 103, 105,
      106, 107, 108
Acetylcholinesterase, 105
Acute leukemia, 25
ADRA (Adventit Development Relief
      Agency), 128
Afghanistan, infant mortality rates, 16-17,
      93
Africa
  consanguineous marriages, 27, 32
  infant mortality rates, 14, 15, 16-17
  prevalence of defects, 28, 29, 32, 98,
      136-137, 144-145, 154-155, 158-
      159, 164-165, 168-171, 174-177,
      184-185, 192-193, 202-203, 206-
      207
  treatment of birth defects, 81-82
African Americans, disorders prevalent
      among, 33
Age factors
  maternal, 4, 6, 24, 26, 71, 95, 99, 103,
      230
  paternal, 103

Albinism. *See* Oculocutaneous albinism
Alcohol-related neurodevelopmental
      disorder, 48-49
Alcohol use during pregnancy
  defects and risks associated with, 4, 36,
      48-49, 52
  interventions, 1, 6, 78-79, 128
Algeria, infant mortality rates, 16, 93
Alpha-fetoprotein blood test, 99, 105, 227
Aminopterin, 36, 45
Amniocentesis, 101, 105, 106-107, 227,
      230
Amniotic fluid, 227
Androgens and androgenic compounds, 35,
      45
Anemia, 41, 231. *See also* Sickle cell disease
  acute hemolytic, 28, 29, 32, 100, 227
Anencephaly, 42, 51, 227
Angiotensin-converting enzyme inhibitors,
      45, 47
Antenatal. *See* Prenatal
Anticholinergic drugs, 45
Anticoagulant drugs, 36, 45, 48, 79
Anticonvulsant drugs, 35, 48, 79
Anti-inflammatory drugs, nonsteroidal, 45
Antimalarial drugs, 32, 100
Antithyroid drugs, 45
Aplasia cutis, 45

Argentina
    monitoring program, 24
    prevalence of defects, 148-149, 182-183,
        196-197, 200-201, 202-203, 208-
        209
Arthrogryposis, 48
Asia
    consanguineous marriages, 27
    immunization programs, 76
    infant mortality rates, 14
    prevalence of defects, 29, 136-139, 144-
        148, 150-151, 154-157, 158-161,
        164-165, 170-171, 176-181, 184-
        187, 192-195, 202-207
Australia, prevalence of defects, 33, 188-189
Autosomal disorders, 11, 27, 34, 227

B

Bahrain
    infant mortality rates, 16-17
    prevalence of defects, 168-169
Bangladesh, school-based rehabilitation
        program, 89, 90
Basic reproductive care, 69-71. *See also*
        Community health programs
    capacity building, 9, 125, 228
    collaborations, 126-128
    data collection, 8, 9, 112
    enhancement strategies, 5-6, 9, 122-128
    and infant mortality, 15
    laboratory standards, 125-126
    primary, 123
    recommendations, 5-6, 9, 71, 112
    secondary, 123-124
    tertiary, 125
    training, 8, 9, 126
Bendectin, 44
Bilirubin encephalopathy, 100, 233
Birth asphyxia, 15
Birth defects. *See also* Birth prevalence of
        defects
    causes and risk factors, 4, 11, 27; *see
        also* Complex birth defects;
        Environmental birth defects;
        Genetic birth defects
    community variability in perceptions and
        expectations, 6
    data accuracy and quality, 14
    defined, 3-4, 11, 228
    global burden of disease, 14

literature sources, 3, 135-211
magnitude of the problem, 12, 14
mortality and morbidity, 11, 15, 233
prevalence, 1, 12, 14, 15, 135-211
social isolation and stigmatization, 86,
        87
Birth prevalence of defects. *See also
        individual countries*
    by country and disorder, 135-211
    defined, 228
    developed countries, 12
    developing countries, 14
    monitoring, 110-111
Blindness. *See* Vision and eye disorders
Blood transfusions and blood product
        safety, 28, 34, 96, 100
Bolivia, prevalence of defects, 196-197,
        208-209
Bone marrow transplantation, 98
Brazil
    prevalence of defects, 31, 48, 140-141,
        148-149, 154-155, 180-181, 186-
        187, 196-197, 202-203, 208-209
    rubella immunization program, 76-77

C

Cameroon, prevalence of defects, 164-165
Canada, prevalence of defects, 23-24, 188-
        189
Cancer, secondary, 45, 86. *See also specific
        types of cancer*
Carbamazepine, 45, 48
Cardiovascular anomalies, 12, 35, 36, 37,
        42, 45, 55
CARE (Cooperative for Assistance and
        Relief Everywhere), 128
Caribbean
    infant mortality rates, 15
    prevalence of defects, 77
Catholic countries, 26
Caucasians, disorders prevalent among, 33,
        34
Central nervous system damage, 35, 36, 40,
        42, 45, 55
Cerebral palsy, 50
Child mortality, 28, 31
Childbirth complications, 15, 50, 78
Chile
    folic acid fortification of foods, 73
    prevalence of defects, 196-197, 208-209

China
  CHD treatment, 85
  folic acid trials for NTDs, 72
  HSV seroprevalence in pregnant women, 41
  monitoring program, 23
  prevalence of defects, 136-137, 150-151, 170-171, 176-177, 184-185, 192-195
Chinese Birth Defects Monitoring Program (CBDMP), 23
Chorionic villus sampling, 101, 105, 106-107, 228
Chorioretinitis, 40, 41
Christmas disease, 34
Chromosomal nondisjunction, 24, 228
Cleft lip and/or cleft palate
  cause and risk factors, 12, 27, 35, 53
  prevalence, 53, 192-201
  signs, symptoms, and sequellae, 52-53, 83-84, 228
  treatment, 83-84
Clinical trials
  effective treatment, 230
  efficacious treatment, 230
  defined, 228
Clubfoot. *See* Talipes
Coagulation factor VIII deficiency, 34
Cocaine, 36
Colombia, prevalence of defects, 196-197, 208-209
Community-based rehabilitation, 83, 87-88, 89, 90, 91, 127, 228-229
Community health programs
  capacity building, 9, 80, 125, 128, 228
  collaborations, 123, 126-128
  data collection, 8, 9, 112, 125
  enhancement strategies, 5-6, 9, 122-128
  genetic screening, 125-126
  incorporation of interventions into existing services, 1, 125, 129-130
  laboratory standards, 125-126
  limiting factors, 17-18, 112
  primary care, 123, 125
  public health campaigns, 128
  recommendations, 5-6, 9, 71, 112
  reproductive health services, 122-128
  secondary care, 123-124
  staffing, 123-124
  tertiary care, 125
  training of workers, 8, 9, 81, 83, 87-88, 90, 102-103, 123, 124-125, 126, 128, 131
Community organizations, 126
Complex birth defects. *See also specific disorders*
  defined, 4, 228
  examples, 13, 51-54
  percentage of all defects, 12
Congenital abnormality, defined, 229
Congenital heart disease (CHD)
  cause and risk factors, 25, 229
  diagnosis, 84
  monitoring infants for, 78
  prevalence, 184-191
  signs, symptoms, and sequellae, 52
  treatment, 84, 85
Congenital hypothyroidism, 43, 45, 108, 229
Congenital infections. *See also specific diseases*
  CMV, 40, 229
  prevention, 1, 4, 76-78
Congenital rubella syndrome, 76-78, 229
  cause and risk factors, 4, 55
  prevalence, 38-40
  prevention, 1, 38, 76-77
  signs, symptoms, and sequellae, 37
  surveillance, 77-78
  survival, 37
Congo, iodine intervention, 74
Consanguineous unions, 4, 27, 31, 32, 33, 34, 103, 128, 229
Constriction rings, 45
Convulsions, 229
Costa Rica
  genetic screening program, 92, 109
  HSV seroprevalence in pregnant women, 41
  infant mortality rate, 92, 93
Coumarin derivatives, 36, 45, 47, 48
Counseling
  genetic, 8, 102-103, 108, 113
  preconceptional, 8, 79, 80, 102-103
  psychological, for families with defects, 84
  recommendations, 79
  training for, 102-103
Craniofacial defects, 36, 45, 48. *See also* Cleft lip and/or cleft palate

Cretinism, 43, 74, 229
Cuba
    genetic screening program, 15, 92, 98,
        99, 104, 109, 129
    infant mortality rates, 18, 92, 93
    prevalence of defects, 31, 140-141, 154-
        155, 166-167
Cyanosis, 229
Cyclophosphamide, 45
Cyprus
    genetic screening program, 15, 104, 109
    infant mortality rates, 16-17
    prevalence of defects, 152-153, 160-161
Cystic fibrosis (CF)
    cause and risk factors, 33
    prevalence, 28, 33-34, 168-169
    screening for, 33, 100, 107
    signs, symptoms, and sequellae, 33, 229-
        230
    survival rates, 230
    treatment, 100
Cytogenetic techniques, 11
Cytomegalovirus (CMV), 35, 39, 40, 229
Czech Republic, prevalence of birth defects,
    170-171

D

Danazol, 45
Dandy-Walker syndrome, 45
Deafness, 35, 36, 37, 40, 41, 43, 50
Developed countries
    maternal age-adjusted risk, 24
    prevalence of defects, 140-143, 148-149,
        152-153, 160-163, 168-169, 180-
        183, 188-191, 198-201, 210-211
Developing countries. *See also individual
        countries*
    burden of disease, 18
    defined, 230
    genetic screening programs, 15-17, 92,
        95, 97-98, 104, 109
    infant mortality rates, 14-15, 18, 93-95
    limiting factors for health services, 17-18
    partnerships with developed countries,
        84, 85
    physicians and nurses, 123, 124
    prevalence of defects, 26
    prevention and care programs for birth
        defects, 2, 82, 85, 87, 88, 90
    public health ministries' role, 6

statistical and registry data, 22
    traditional health focus, 9
Developmental dysplasia of the hip
    cause and risk factors, 12, 54, 230
    diagnosis, 54, 84, 108
    prevalence, 54, 206-211
    screening for, 108
    signs, symptoms, and sequellae, 230
    treatment or correction of, 54, 84-86, 108
Dhaka University, 90
Diabetes. *See* Insulin-dependent diabetes
        mellitus
Diagnostic radiography, 50-51
Diazepan, 44
Diethylstilbestrol, 36, 45
Disability-adjusted life years (DALY)
        measure, 127
Down syndrome
    cause and risk factors, 24, 26, 52, 55,
        71, 228, 230
    prevalence, 26, 144-149
    prevention, 1, 6, 71
    screening and detection, 105, 106, 111,
        227, 228, 230
    signs, symptoms, and sequellae, 25-26,
        52, 230
    survival, 26
Drugs. *See* Medications; Recreational drugs
Dysarthria, 50

E

Eastern Europe, prevalence of defects, 138-
        141, 150-151, 160-161, 168-173,
        206-207. *See also individual
        countries*
Ebstein's anomaly, 36, 45
Echocardiography, 46, 47, 52
Education programs, 5, 6, 71, 79, 86, 89,
        102, 125, 126, 132
Egypt
    infant mortality rates, 16-17, 93
    prevalence of defects, 184-185
    toxoplasmosis seroprevalence in
        pregnant women, 40
Encephalocele, 42, 51, 230
Environmental birth defects. *See also*
        Complex birth defects;
        Teratogens
    alcohol and recreational drug use, 4, 48-
        50

causes and risk factors, 4, 11, 13, 37-49;
    see also specific causes
defined, 230
examples of, 13
infectious pathogens, 4, 37-41
interventions, 71-80
maternal health and nutrition and, 42
percentage of all birth defects, 11
pollutants, 4, 50, 79
radiation, 50-51
Environmental pollutants, 8, 50, 79, 128
Epidemiological data
    large-scale monitoring programs, 23, 24
    quality and completeness of, 14, 110
    recommendations on collection of, 8-9,
        110-111, 125, 132, 133
    sources for this study, 19
Epiphyseal stippling, 36, 48
Ergotamine, 46
Eritrea, HSV seroprevalence in pregnant
    women, 41
Estonia, prevalence of defects, 101, 170-171
Ethical considerations, 108-109
Ethiopia
    CHD treatment, 85
    infant mortality rates, 16-17, 93
Ethnic origin, and prevalence of disorders,
    31, 33, 54, 103
European Register of Congenital
    Abnormalities and Twins
    (EUROCAT), 23
Eye. *See* Vision and eye disorders

F

Failure to thrive, 29
Family planning, 5, 55, 69, 71, 79, 104,
    123, 128
Fertility rates, 18
Fetal alcohol syndrome
    cause and risk factors, 48-49, 55, 78
    prevalence, 49
    prevention, 78-79
    signs, symptoms, and sequellae, 49, 78,
        231
Fetal karyotyping, 84, 106, 107
Fetal ultrasonography, 46, 47, 99, 105-106,
    231
Finland, prevalence of defects, 188-189
Fogarty International Center Training and
    Research Programs, 133

Folic acid
    antagonists, 36
    deficiency, 1, 4, 42, 52, 55, 227
    dietary sources, 72
    fortification of foods, 1, 6, 71-73
    supplementation, 70, 71-72, 98, 128

G

Gambia, cytomegalovirus immunity in
    women, 40
Genetic birth defects. *See also* Complex
    birth defects; Screening for
    genetic disorders; *individual*
    disorders
    carriers, 28, 31, 32, 228, 231
    chromosomal disorders, 4, 13, 23-26,
        52, 103, 107, 227, 228
    counseling about risk, 102-103
    defined, 11, 231
    detection, 11
    dominant traits, 11, 230
    examples of, 13
    maternal age and, 4, 6, 24, 26, 230
    percentage of all birth defects, 11
    single-gene disorders, 4, 11-12, 13, 27-
        34, 105, 107
Genetic histories, 103
Genital anomalies, 35, 36, 45
Genital herpes, 41, 78
Germany, prevalence of defects, 23-24
Global Burden of Disease Study,
    127-128
Glucose-6-phosphate dehydrogenase
    (G6PD) deficiency
    cause and risk factors, 28, 32
    geographic distribution, 32
    interventions, 99-100
    malaria resistance in carriers, 32
    prevalence, by country, 158-163
    screening for, 95, 99-100, 107-108
    signs, symptoms, and sequellae, 99, 100,
        231
Goiter, 43, 45, 231
Goitrogens, 74
Greece
    genetic screening and control program,
        97, 104, 109
    prevalence of defects, 97, 162-163
Growth retardation, 26, 34, 41, 45, 48

H

Haiti, HSV seroprevalence in pregnant
    women, 41
Hb H disease, 28-29
Health care services. *See also* Basic
    reproductive care; Community
    health programs; Treatment of
    birth defects; *specific services*
  coordination of, 5, 8, 111-112, 130-131
  evidence-based care, 230-231
  Internet communication, 8-9, 131-132
  monitoring health care delivery and
    outcomes, 81, 131
  national policy and leadership, 5, 111-
    112, 129-133
  priority setting, 81, 131
  recommendations, 7, 8-9, 80, 91
  research, 90, 125, 132-133
  strategies for addressing birth defects,
    122-129
  terminal and palliative, 91
Hemarthrosis, 102
Hemolysis, 231
Hemophilias A and B
  cause and risk factors, 34, 102, 232
  prevalence, 28, 34
  screening for, 101-102
  signs, symptoms, and sequellae, 34, 232
  treatment, 102
Heparin, 47, 48, 79
Hepatitis B, 34, 102
Hepatomegaly, 28, 41, 232
Herpes simplex virus (HSV), 35, 39, 41, 78
Heterozygotes, 28, 232
HIV/AIDS, 14, 34, 44, 102
Holoprosencephaly, 232
Homozygotes, 28, 232
Hong Kong, prevalence of defects, 152-153,
    162-163, 210-211
Hospital admissions and lengths of stay, 15
Human chorionic gonadotropin, 105
Hungary, prevalence of defects, 138-141,
    206-207
Hydraencephaly, 232
Hydrocephalus
  causes and risk factors, 41, 45, 48, 51
  defined, 232
  prevalence, 174-183
Hydroxyurea, 98

Hyperbilirubinemia, 100, 232
Hyperthermia, 42, 232
Hypoglycemic drugs, 45, 46
Hypothyroidism. *See* Congenital
    hypothyroidism

I

Immunization programs, 6, 76-78, 127. *See
    also* Vaccines
India
  consanguineous marriages, 27
  folic acid trials for NTDs, 72
  HSV seroprevalence in pregnant women,
    41
  intervention programs, 82, 102
  prevalence of defects, 27, 29, 31, 39, 99,
    138-139, 146-147, 150-151, 154-
    161, 178-181, 184-187, 194-195,
    204-205, 206-207
  privatization of health services, 126
  rubella susceptibility in pregnant
    women, 39
Indonesia
  prevalence of defects, 136-137, 146-147,
    164-165, 176-177, 184-185, 194-
    195, 204-205
  toxoplasmosis seroprevalence in
    pregnant women, 40
Infant mortality rates, 5, 14-15, 26, 27, 37,
    92
  by country, 93-95
  defined, 232
Infectious agents. *See also* Congenital
    infections; *specific agents*
  defects and risks associated with, 35, 36,
    37
  diagnostic difficulties, 37
  prevention of defects from, 37, 78, 128
  teratogenic pathogens, 4, 37-41
Inhibin A, 105
Insulin-dependent diabetes mellitus (IDDM),
    35, 42, 52, 55, 232-233
International agencies, 123, 127
International Clearinghouse for Birth
    Defects Monitoring System
    (ICBDMS), 23
International Clinical Epidemiology
    Network, 133

Intervention strategies, 112-113. *See also* Basic reproductive care; Rehabilitation; Treatment of birth defects
alcohol avoidance during pregnancy, 78-79
cost-effectiveness analysis, 81, 106, 132, 229
determinants of success, 6, 69
identification of risk factors, 70
incorporation into existing services, 129-130
low-cost preventive strategies, 1, 5-6, 42, 71-80
national coordination of, 5, 76, 79, 110-112
recommendations, 5-7, 7-9, 71, 73, 76, 78, 79, 80
regulatory, 79
rehabilitation-related, 87-92
staging process, 68, 92, 112-113
surveillance and monitoring, 5, 110-112
Intracranial calcification, 41, 233
Intrauterine growth retardation, 50
Iodine
assessment of nutritional status, 73-74
distribution of households by iodized salt use, 75
goitrogen interference with, 74
intramuscular injection of fortified oil, 74
population with inadequate intakes, 74
recommendation, 76
salt fortification, 1, 6, 74-76
Iodine deficiency disorders
cause and risk factors, 36, 43, 55, 73, 233
prevalence, 43
prevention, 1, 6, 73-76
signs, symptoms, and sequellae, 1, 43-44, 229, 233
Ionizing radiation, 36, 50-51
Iran
genetic screening program, 15, 97, 104, 109, 129, 130
infant mortality rates, 16-17, 94
prevalence of defects, 170-171, 196-197
Iraq
infant mortality rates, 16-17, 94
methylmercury poisoning, 50
prevalence of defects, 160-161

Ireland, prevalence of defects, 26
Isotretinoin, 46
Israel
prevalence of defects, 39, 148-149, 168-169, 182-183, 190-191, 198-199, 210-211
rubella susceptibility in pregnant women, 39
Save a Child's Heart Foundation, 84, 85
Wolfson Medical Center, 85
Italy
HSV seroprevalence in pregnant women, 41
prevalence of defects, 26, 140-141, 182-183, 188-189, 198-199
Ivory Coast
cytomegalovirus immunity in women, 40
prevalence of defects, 40

J

Jamaica
HSV seroprevalence in pregnant women, 41
prevalence of defects, 39
rubella susceptibility in pregnant women, 39
3D Projects, 87, 88
Japan
HSV seroprevalence in pregnant women, 41
methylmercury poisoning, 50
prevalence of defects, 33, 54, 140-141, 198-199
traditional infant care practices, 54
Jaundice, 41, 107, 233
hemolytic, 32, 231-232
Jordan
infant mortality rates, 16-17, 94
prevalence of defects, 33, 150-151, 156-157, 168-169, 180-181

K

Kernicterus, 32, 107, 233
Kuwait
infant mortality rates, 16-17
prevalence of defects, 148-149

L

Lapps, traditional infant care practices, 54
Latin America. *See also individual countries*
   genetic screening, 5, 100
   immunization programs, 76
   infant mortality rates, 5, 15
   prevalence of defects, 33, 77, 100, 140-
      141, 148-149, 154-155, 166-167,
      180-181, 186-187, 196-199, 202-
      203, 208-209
   privatization of health services, 126
Latin American Collaborative Study of
      Congenital Malformations
      (ECLAMC), 23, 24
Latvia, prevalence of birth defects, 101,
      172-173
Lebanon
   infant mortality rates, 16-17, 94
   prevalence of defects, 140-141, 208-209
Leprosy, 44
Lethal traits, 11, 28, 111
Libya
   infant mortality rates, 16-17, 94
   prevalence of defects, 144-145, 158-159
Limb reduction deformities, 36, 42, 44, 45,
      48, 234
Literacy, 18, 69
Lithium, 36, 45, 46, 47
Low birth weight, 15, 101, 233

M

Macrosomia, 233
Malaria resistance in carriers, 28, 231
Malaysia
   prevalence of defects, 39, 136-137, 144-
      145, 158-159, 202-203, 206-207
   rubella susceptibility in pregnant
      women, 39
March of Dimes, 128
Maternal risk factors
   age over 35 years, 4, 6, 24, 26, 71, 95,
      99, 103, 230
   alcohol abuse, 4, 36, 48-49, 52, 55
   educational status, 69
   epilepsy polytherapy, 48, 79
   IDDM, 35, 42, 52, 55
   infectious agents, 37, 38-39, 40, 41, 52
   medications, 44-48
   nutritional deficiencies, 4, 6, 42-44

   occupational exposures to pollutants,
      50, 79
   phenylketonuria, 35, 42
   public education campaigns, 128
   screening for, 95, 99, 105
Medical Group Mission Christian Medical
      and Dental Society, 83
Medications
   defects and risks associated with, 35-36,
      44-45, 48
   oxidant drugs, 32, 100
   public education campaigns, 128
   safe for pregnant women, 44, 46-47
   teratogenic, 4, 6, 35-36, 44-45, 48, 79-
      80, 128
Meningoencephalitis, 233
Mental retardation, 1, 2, 11, 23, 26, 34, 37,
      40, 41, 43-44, 48, 49, 50, 101,
      108, 230, 231
Methimazole, 45
Methotrexate, 36, 45
Methylmercury, 6, 36, 50, 79
Microcephaly, 34, 35, 36, 41, 48, 78
Microthalmia, 78
Microtia-anotia, 36
Middle East. *See also individual countries*
   consanguineous marriages, 27
   genetic screening, 5
   infant mortality rates, 5, 15, 16-17
   prevalence of defects, 29, 138-141, 146-
      147, 150-151, 156-157, 160-161,
      168-171, 180-181, 186-187, 194-
      197, 206-209
Misoprostol (RU-486), 45, 48, 79
Moebius sequence, 45
Moldova, CHD treatment, 85
Monitoring birth defects. *See* Surveillance
      and monitoring
Morocco, infant mortality rates, 16-17,
      94
Mothballs, 32
Myelomenigocele, 233
Myxedema, 43, 233

N

Naphthalene, 32
Nasal hypoplasia, 36, 48
National Institutes of Health (U.S.), 133
National policy and leadership roles
   coordination of services, 130-131

incorporating interventions into existing
  programs, 129-130
Internet site, 8-9, 131-132
monitoring health care delivery and
  outcomes, 81, 131
priority setting, 131
recommendations, 8-9, 111-112
research capacity building, 132-133
training standards, 131
Native Americans, traditional infant care
  practices, 54
Necrotizing enterocolitis, 45
Neonatal
  care, 70-71
  hypoglycemia, 45
  meconium ileus, 45
  screening for genetic disorders, 5, 107-
    108
  withdrawal syndrome, 45
Neural tube defects
  cause and risk factors, 27, 42, 45, 48,
    52, 71, 233-234
  prevalence, 42, 51-52, 174-183
  prevention, 1, 6, 47, 52, 70, 71-73
  screening for, 52, 99, 105, 106, 111,
    227
  signs, symptoms, and sequellae, 51-52
  treatment, 51
  types, 51-52
Neurological damage and disorders, 35, 36,
    40, 42, 43
NGO Networks for Health, 128
Niger, infant mortality rates, 18, 94
Nigeria
  CHD treatment, 85
  mortality from defects, 33
  prevalence of defects, 31, 33, 39, 144-
    145, 154-155, 164-165, 176-177
  rubella susceptibility in pregnant
    women, 39
  toxoplasmosis seroprevalence in
    pregnant women, 41
Nongovernmental organizations (NGOs),
    123, 126, 127, 128
Nystagmus, 33

O

Oculocutaneous albinism
  cause and risk factors, 32-33, 234
  geographic distribution, 28, 33

myths and superstitions, 86
prevalence, 164-167
screening for, 111
signs, symptoms, and sequellae, 33, 86,
    234
treatment, 86-87
Oman
  infant mortality rates, 16-17
  prevalence of defects, 39, 186-187
  rubella susceptibility in pregnant
    women, 39
Operation Smile, 83
Oral contraceptives, 44
Ortolani-Barlow test, 84

P

Pacific Islands, prevalence of birth defects,
    29
Pakistan
  infant mortality rates, 16-17, 94
  prevalence of defects, 146-147, 154-155,
    158-159, 176-177, 184-185, 206-
    207
Palestine National Authority
  CHD treatment, 85
  consanguineous marriages, 27
  infant mortality rates, 16-17, 27
Panama
  prevalence of defects, 39
  rubella susceptibility in pregnant
    women, 39
Papua New Guinea, prevalence of birth
    defects, 29
Paramethadione, 45
Patent ductus arteriosus, 39, 45
PATH (Program for Appropriate
    Technology in Health), 128
Peru, prevalence of defects, 196-197, 208-
    209
Phenobarbital, 48
Phenylalanine hydroxylase, 34
Phenylketonuria
  cause and risk factors, 34, 35, 42, 234
  prevalence in neonates, 28, 34, 101,
    170-173
  screening for, 2, 96, 99, 100-101, 108
  signs, symptoms, and sequellae, 34, 101,
    234
  treatment, 42, 101, 108
Phenylpyruvale, 34

Phenytoin, 45, 48
Philippines, prevalence of birth defects, 192-193
Photophobia, 33, 234
Pigmentation disorders, 32-33, 34
Placental biopsy, 101
Plan International, 128
Poland, prevalence of birth defects, 170-171
Pollutants. *See* Environmental pollutants
Population and Family Planning Expansion Project, 128
Preconceptional care, 5, 69-70
Pregnancy. *See also* Maternal risk factors
    diagnostic radiography, 50-51
    prevention in women over 35, 71
    safe medications, 44, 46-47, 48, 79
Prenatal care
    educational campaigns, 5
    screening and diagnosis of defects, 2, 5, 70, 80, 95, 97-98, 105-107
Prevalence of birth defects. *See also* Birth prevalence of defects
    defined, 234
    determinants, 22, 24
Primaquine, 32
Professional societies, 127, 128
Propylthiouracil, 45
Protibondhi Foundation, 89
Psychoactive drugs, 45
Psychomotor retardation, 40
Public health educational campaigns, 6, 7, 79, 86, 112, 128, 130
Purpose of this study, 18-19

Q

Qatar, infant mortality rates, 16-17

R

Radiation. *See* Ionizing radiation
Recommendations
    basic reproductive care, 5-6, 9, 71
    cost-effective interventions, 4, 5-7, 71, 73, 76, 78, 79, 80
    education policies, 91
    genetic screening programs, 7-8, 110
    health care improvements for infants, 7, 87, 91
    national coordination, surveillance, and monitoring, 8-9, 111-112

Recreational drugs, defects and risks associated with, 36
Rehabilitation
    community-based, 83, 87-88, 89, 90, 91, 127, 228-229
    institutional and hospital-based care, 90-91, 102
    primary health care model, 91
    psychosocial support for families, 7, 84, 92, 127
    and quality of life, 71
    recommendations, 7, 132
    research, 132
    school-based models, 7, 89, 90, 127
    villages, 90
Renal defects, 42, 45
Reproductive care. *See* Basic reproductive care
Research agenda, 132-133
Retinoids, systemic, 36, 45, 79
Risk factors. *See also* Maternal risk factors; *individual birth defects*
    identification of risk factors, 70
Rubella. *See also* Congenital rubella syndrome
    defects and risk associated with, 35, 37, 52
    immunization against, 1, 4, 6, 38, 76-78
    incidence, 38
    maternal immunity, 38
    screening for, 39, 78
    susceptibility in pregnant women, 39
Rwanda, HSV seroprevalence in pregnant women, 41

S

Salicylates, 44
Sardinia
    genetic screening and control program, 97, 104, 109
    prevalence of defects, 97, 152-153
Saudi Arabia
    consanguineous marriages, 27
    infant mortality rates, 16-17, 95
    prevalence of birth defects, 27, 31, 54, 146-147, 156-157, 180-181, 194-197, 206-207
    traditional infant care practices, 54
Save a Child's Heart Foundation, 84, 85
Save the Children, 127, 128, 133

Screening for genetic disorders
components of, 109
counseling, 8, 98, 99, 102-103, 109, 113
criteria for establishing programs, 68,
96-102
defined, 231
ethical considerations, 108-109, 130
examples of national programs, 15-17,
92, 95, 97-98, 109, 111, 129
introducing services for, 109, 125, 129
neonatal, 2, 5, 95, 107-108, 129
pilot programs, 106
preconceptional, 2, 4, 95, 97, 98, 103-
104, 129
prenatal diagnosis, 2, 5, 80, 95, 97-98,
101, 105-107, 129
purpose of, 92, 95, 113
recommendations, 4-5, 7-9, 110
Screening for infectious diseases, 39
Seizure disorder, 41, 229, 235
Senegal, HSV seroprevalence in pregnant
women, 41
Sexual differentiation disorders, 23, 45
Sickle cell disease
cause and risk factors, 30, 31, 235
geographic distribution, 30, 31, 235
prevalence, 31, 154-157
prevention, 99
malaria resistance in carriers, 28, 31,
231
screening for, 95, 96, 98-99, 104, 107
signs, symptoms, and sequellae, 30-31,
98, 99, 235
treatment, 98
Sierra Leone, prevalence of defects, 154-155
Singapore
prevalence of defects, 39, 160-161, 198-
199
rubella susceptibility in pregnant
women, 39
Skin disorders, 34, 35, 86
Somalia, infant mortality rates, 16, 95
South Africa
cytomegalovirus immunity in women, 40
genetic screening program, 15, 109, 111,
129
prevalence of defects, 26, 33, 40, 49,
101, 111, 136-137, 144-145,
164-165, 170-171, 174-175, 184-
185, 192-193, 202-203

South America. *See also* Latin America,
individual countries
prevalence of defects, 26, 44, 198-199,
202-203, 208-209
South Korea
cytomegalovirus immunity in women, 40
prevalence of defects, 140-141, 182-183,
188-189, 210-211
Southeast Asia, prevalence of defects, 29.
See also individual countries
Spain
HSV seroprevalence in pregnant women,
41
prevalence of defects, 196-197
Spermicides, 44
Spina bifida, 35, 42, 51, 53, 227, 235
Splenomegaly, 28, 29, 41, 235
Squamous cell carcinoma, 32-33, 235
Sri Lanka
prevalence of defects, 39
rubella susceptibility in pregnant
women, 39
Stem cell transplant, 96-97
Stillbirths, 26, 27, 103, 111, 235
Streptococcus pneumoniae, 31
Streptokinase, 47
Sub-Saharan Africa. *See also individual
countries*
genetic birth defects, 31
infant mortality rates, 14
Sudan, infant mortality rates, 16-17, 95
Sulfonamide antibiotics and sulfones, 32
Support services for families, 7
Surveillance and monitoring
defined, 235
of delivery of health services and
treatment outcomes, 81, 131
large-scale programs, 23, 24
national coordination of, 5, 110-112
of rubella and CRS, 77-78
Sweden, prevalence of defects, 198-199
Syria, infant mortality rates, 16-17, 95

T

Taiwan
HSV seroprevalence in pregnant women,
41
prevalence of defects, 158-159
Talipes or clubfoot
cause and risk factors, 53, 107

prevalence, 53, 202-205
signs, symptoms, and sequellae, 53, 235
treatment, 81-83
Tanzania
  CHD treatment, 85
  mortality from defects, 33
  prevalence of defects, 176-177
  talipes treatment program, 82
  toxoplasmosis seroprevalence in
    pregnant women, 40-41
Teratogens. See also Environmental birth
    defects
  defects and risk factors, 35-36
  defined, 235-236
  determinants of damage by, 35
  regulation of occupational exposures, 6
Tetracycline, 45
Thailand
  cytomegalovirus immunity in women, 40
  genetic screening program, 98
  prevalence of defects, 39, 150-151, 158-
    159, 184-185, 204-205
  rubella susceptibility in pregnant
    women, 39
  toxoplasmosis seroprevalence in
    pregnant women, 40
Thalassemias
  cause and risk factors, 28, 236
  geographic distribution, 29-30
  malaria resistance in carriers, 28
  prevalence, 28, 150-153
  screening for, 95, 96-98, 104, 107, 109,
    130
  signs, symptoms, and sequellae, 28-29,
    236
  treatment, 28, 96-97, 130
Thalidomide, 36, 44, 45, 79
3D Projects, 87, 88
Thymic defects, 36
Toxoplasma gondii, 40-41
Toxoplasmosis, 35, 39, 40-41, 78, 236
Treatment of birth defects. See also
    Rehabilitation
  access to, 80
  comprehensive, 84
  early diagnosis and, 7, 70, 80, 83, 100
  parental education component, 82
  recommendations, 7
  screening and referral, 80
Trimethadione, 45

Trinidad and Tobago
  prevalence of defects, 39
  rubella susceptibility in pregnant
    women, 39
Trisomy 13, 24, 26, 71, 236
Trisomy 18, 24, 26, 71, 236
Trisomy 21. See Down Syndrome
Tunisia
  infant mortality rates, 16-17, 95
  prevalence of birth defects, 33, 136-137,
    174-175, 184-185, 192-193, 202-
    203, 206-207
Turkey
  cytomegalovirus immunity in women, 40
  prevalence of defects, 34, 54, 142-143,
    150-151, 160-161, 168-169, 172-
    173
  screening and control programs, 97-98,
    102
  traditional infant care practices, 54
Tyrosinase, 32, 34

U

Uganda, prevalence of birth defects, 136-
    137, 192-193, 202-203
Ultrasonography, 46, 47, 84-85, 99, 105-
    106, 107, 231, 236
Unconjugated estriol, 105
United Arab Emirates
  consanguineous marriages, 27
  infant mortality rates, 16-17
  prevalence of birth defects, 27, 138-139
United Kingdom
  folic acid fortification of foods, 73
  prevalence of defects, 26, 180-181
United Nations Children's Fund, 127
United Nations Development Programme,
    127
United Nations Educational, Scientific and
    Cultural Organization
    Declaration of Education for All,
    89
United States
  folic acid fortification of foods, 73
  prevalence of defects, 23-24, 140-141,
    180-181, 188-189, 198-199
Urinary tract defects, 36, 45
U.S. Agency for International Development,
    128

V

Vaccines. *See also* Immunization programs
  fetal risk, 77
  measles-mumps-rubella (MMR), 76, 77
Vaginal carcinoma, 45
Valproic acid, 45, 47, 48
Venezuela, prevalence of birth defects, 196-
  197, 208-209
Vision and eye disorders, 33, 35, 37, 39,
  40, 41, 43, 48, 50, 78, 234
Vitamin A deficiency, 74

W

Warfarin, 45, 47, 48
World Atlas of Birth Defects, 23
World Bank, 127
World Health Organization, 87-88, 127
  Special Programme for Research and
    Training on Tropical Diseases,
    133
World Summit for Children, 74

X

X-linked disorders, 27, 32, 34, 237

Y

Yemen, infant mortality rates, 16-17, 95

Z

Zaire
  HSV seroprevalence in pregnant women,
    41
  prevalence of defects, 192-193
Zambia, "clubfoot clinic," 82
Zimbabwe
  prevalence of defects, 33, 136-137, 164-
    165, 174-175, 192-193
  rehabilitation approaches, 86, 89, 91